ADVANCE PRAISE FOR SOMETHING DEEPER

"Tom Hudson's *Something Deeper* is a profound exploration of the interconnectedness of all things. It presents a compelling argument for integrating spirituality into our everyday existence. With wisdom and eloquence, Hudson guides readers on a transformative journey, teaching them how to tap into incredible value and meaning found even in the most mundane moments. This book is not just a thought-provoking read; it's a life-affirming guide for anyone looking to live a more fulfilled and connected life."

—**DAVID PERLMUTTER**, MD, No. 1 New York Times Bestselling Author of *Grain Brain*

"Tom Hudson takes us on a healing journey to find the magic in everyday life. There's wisdom in these pages that will keep you on the path to wholeness. Choose to dive deep into this book now and enrich your life in unexpected ways!"

—**LARRY BURK**, MD, CEHP, Author of *Let Magic Happen: Adventures in Healing with a Holistic Radiologist*

"This is one of the most meaningful books I've read in years. Dr. Tom Hudson takes the reader on a journey to discover how to connect the deeper aspects of life to everyday living. He reminds us that life is meant to be lived fully and attuned to the beauty of each day. I highly recommend this book to anyone feeling stuck in the mundane. Treat yourself to 31 days of self-discovery that will transform your thinking and fill you with great joy."

—**JOANNE ELLISON**, Founder, Drawing Near to God Ministry

"*Something Deeper* is much more than a collection of poems; it is a timely and important opportunity to counter the uncertainties of life today. These are gentle teachings written from the heart – a humble offering of personal experience for your own journey towards enlightenment through a deeper understanding of your own emotions, thoughts, fears, joys, and heartaches. Everyone can identify with the poignant message in each poem. It is very personal, and it "resonates" as you travel through each daily reading, realizing just how powerful they are. Dr. Hudson gives you the formulas to put your newfound understanding and wisdom into daily practice! You will feel "connected." Readers will be profoundly moved by this book… and the better for it."

—**PETER LEANDO**, PhD, DSc(Med), DAc
Fellow, Royal Society of Medicine
Founder, Meditherm Inc.

"*Something Deeper* is a captivating and spiritually enlightening book that takes readers on a transformative journey of self-reflection. With its evocative prose and thought-provoking themes, each daily entry provides a profound exploration of human emotions, spirituality, and the complexities of life. The book's well-structured format allows for a mindful and intentional reading experience, making it an ideal companion for personal reflection and meditation. Something Deeper serves as an invaluable resource for individuals seeking solace, inspiration, and a deeper understanding of themselves and the world around them."

—**AKYIAA AZULA**, AP, OMD,
Founder, Creation for Manifesting Miracles

"As to be expected, Dr. Tom Hudson's book, *Something Deeper*, invites us to look at our seemingly ordinary lives and find the hidden lessons to savor. Comprising 31 spiritual poems or devotionals about simple things – those we often overlook or ignore due to busyness and distractions – this book calls us to go beneath the surface and ponder deeper meanings. For those flying through life and wondering how it passes so quickly, this treasure trove of poems helps us slow down and realize there is more... so much more. You'll find yourself returning to these reflections often."

—**CATHEE POULSEN**, Author of *Thresholds and Passages* and *Quiet Places*

SOMETHING DEEPER

SOMETHING DEEPER

31 Spiritual Poems to Help You Navigate Life

Thomas Hudson, M.D.

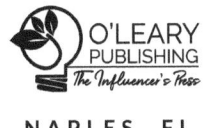

NAPLES, FL

Copyright © 2024 by Thomas Hudson, M.D.
All rights reserved.

Published in the United States by
O'Leary Publishing
www.olearypublishing.com

The views, information, or opinions expressed in this book are solely those of the authors involved and do not necessarily represent those of O'Leary Publishing, LLC.

The author has made every effort possible to ensure the accuracy of the information presented in this book. However, the information herein is sold without warranty, either expressed or implied. Neither the author, publisher, nor any dealer or distributor of this book will be held liable for any damages caused either directly or indirectly by the instructions or information contained in this book. You are encouraged to seek professional advice before taking any action mentioned herein.

All rights reserved. No part of this book may be reproduced or transmitted in any form by any means, electronic, mechanical, photocopy, recording, or other without the prior and express written permission of the author, except for brief cited quotes. For information on getting permission for reprints and excerpts, contact: O'Leary Publishing.

ISBN: print 978-1-952491-59-7
ISBN: eBook 978-1-952491-61-0
Library of Congress: 2023914506

Developmental Editing by Heather Davis Desrocher
Line Editing by Kat Langenheim
Proofreading by Boris Boland
Cover and interior design by Jessica Angerstein
Cover Art by Abigail Orr
Printed in the United States of America

About the Cover

As I thought about the cover for *Something Deeper*, I had a certain look in mind. On a whim, I shared my idea with Abigail, the ten-year old daughter of a close friend. Abigail is creative and quite intuitive, and I had the feeling she would "get" my vision. I thought I could use what she created to give the cover designers an idea of what I wanted. Well, to my surprise, she came up with a beautiful painting that captured exactly what I had envisioned. The final cover is her painting with a few minor tweaks. So, thank you, Abigail. You are more talented than you know!

To Mom and Dad

Know what is in front of your face, and what is hidden from you will be disclosed to you. For there is nothing hidden that won't be revealed.

—GOSPEL OF THOMAS

Contents

Preface i
Introduction 1

Day 1   The Ladder of Life 7
Day 2   Returning Home 13
Day 3   A Long and Winding Road 19
Day 4   The Last Drop 25
Day 5   A Peaceful Evening 31
Day 6   A Mundane Day 36
Day 7   The Placebo Effect 41
Day 8   A Boy and His Dog 46
Day 9   Grateful 54
Day 10 The Pizza Guy 57
Day 11 An Old Friend 65
Day 12 Dare to Dream 70
Day 13 A Home Far Away 75
Day 14 An Off Day 82
Day 15 No Place Like Home 87
Day 16 What Will They Say? 91
Day 17 Precious Moments 96
Day 18 Anonymous 100
Day 19 Mistakes 104

Day 20	Hi, Mom!	108
Day 21	An Opportunity	111
Day 22	Frustrated	118
Day 23	Am I Smiling?	123
Day 24	A Troubling Memory	128
Day 25	Disappointed	133
Day 26	A Long Overdue Goodbye	138
Day 27	The Magic Flute	143
Day 28	The Inner Critic	149
Day 29	Graduation Day	156
Day 30	The Rest of the Time	163
Day 31	A Labor of Love	168

Conclusion	171
Putting it All Together	173
Going Deeper	177
A Parting Gift	210
Acknowledgments	213
About the Author	215

Preface

*Tell people there is an invisible man in the sky who
created the universe, and the vast majority will believe you.
Tell them the paint is wet, and they have to touch it to be sure.*

—GEORGE CARLIN

There is deep truth in this lighthearted quote by George Carlin – that profound truths can be found in the simplest of things. In fact, the quote points out one of the main dilemmas of modern life: the internal disconnect most of us have between the deeper things of life (the man in the sky), and so-called everyday events (the wet paint). It's a disconnect I've felt all my life. And I know I'm not alone.

Even having had many deep spiritual experiences, I'm always amazed how easy it is to go back to "normal life," acting as if they had never happened. I mean, how is that even possible? And yet, it happens all the time. I've tried church, meditation and prayer groups, spiritual books, and intuition classes, just to name a few. And I have loved them all. Each has added to the depth of my experience; they just haven't helped me keep an everyday awareness of that depth.

But if everything in the universe is interconnected (and it is), then I should be able to find that depth any*where*, in any*thing*. I should be able to look at any object, or observe any event, on any given day, and find a deeper meaning.

So, inspired by a "random" comment by my yoga teacher, I began to pay more attention – and that changed everything. I realized I'd been looking at it all wrong. Spirit can't be compartmentalized in a building, or a class, or a great book. *Everyday life* is church. *Everyday life* is spiritual practice. *Everyday life* can be our path to wholeness. But we'll never see it as long as we equate "everyday" with "boring," which it is most definitely not.

This book is for those who want a deeper experience of life, and to have it more consistently. It's for those who have a nagging sense that there's more to life, but aren't quite sure where to look for it. *Something Deeper* is meant to help you experience Spirit in an ongoing, everyday, non-religious way, and to give you a glimpse of how life *really* works, instead of how we always thought it worked. It is so much simpler than we thought. And the best thing is, we don't have to go anywhere to find it. In any given moment, of any given day, all we have to do is look around us – because it's right there, and always has been.

> *Sometimes the simplest things*
> *are the most profound.*
>
> —CAROLINA HERRERA

Introduction
Every Journey Is Inward

How long does it take to write a book? Well, it depends on the book, of course. But for some books, like this one, you have to live it first, which can take a very long time. Sometimes even a lifetime.

Looking back, I've had an intense curiosity for my whole life about how things work – just not in a mechanical kind of way. I could not care any less how a clock works, as long as it tells time. I'm glad *somebody* does, of course. I'm just glad it doesn't have to be me. But I have always been fascinated with how the universe works, how the world works as part of that universe, and how we humans function as part of the overall framework – because, at the end of the day, it's all such a mystery.

It only takes a cursory investigation into any subject to realize how interconnected everything is. And it is just that understanding, I've come to believe, that largely determines our experience of life. When I am aware of the connection on a day-to-day basis, my life is full of awe, and wonder, and gratitude. But when I settle for a surface-only, material view of things, I miss all of that. And that's a pretty big loss.

The more I consider things, the more I believe that awe, and wonder, and gratitude are how we were designed to function. Admittedly, the only evidence I can come up with for this is that they feel so darn good. But isn't that evidence enough? Do we really need a controlled study, as if one could ever be designed for such things?

So, why then, if awe, wonder, and gratitude are part of our operating system, are they absent so much of the time? If they are so beneficial, wouldn't any competent designer make it so that we experience them all the time, no matter what? I can't say I have a definite answer to that one, other than there's the "free will" issue to consider. Yes, perhaps we have to *choose* them. And we choose them, or not, by how we decide to look at life.

I'm not exactly sure when the great divide between the material and non-material realms happened in Western culture. Such a separation does not exist in Eastern cultures. Some say it was in the early 1600s, when the Pope gave Rene Descartes his blessing to dissect human cadavers, as long as Descartes agreed that the soul was separate from the physical body. "The body can belong to science," he was reportedly told, "but the soul belongs to *us*." The deeper message, of course, was, "You're free to do what you want, as long as you keep your hands off our stuff." Descartes took the deal, and was then free to work on his cadavers without fear of being burned at the stake.

If true, it was an expedient deal for him, and I can see why he was happy to make it. But if that's where the separation occurred, anatomic science's short-term gain was Western culture's massive long-term loss, because the beautiful and delicate connection between the surface material world and the deeper mystery beneath it was severed. And the wonder was lost – and the awe, and the gratitude along with it.

It isn't a science versus spirit issue. As science has evolved, it has made the interconnection and the mystery even more evident. The experts on quantum physics have no idea how it all really works, and they'd be the first to tell you that. Thus, even though science now completely agrees that a material-only view of the world is wholly inadequate, the mindset persists in the culture – to all of our detriment, I would submit.

And, even though I've always been fascinated by that deeper connection, there's something about decades of education based in a surface-only paradigm, and a long career in a field mired in the same point of view, that tends to make one forget. Oh, we all know on a deeper level that there's a larger mystery; but our involvement in the culture, which can hardly be avoided, tends to draw our attention elsewhere.

It's kind of like ice skating on a lake, thinking that the ice is all there is, while ignoring an entire ecosystem just inches below, treating it as if it doesn't exist. It sounds ludicrous, yes. But it's what most of us do most of the time. The whole trick of life then, if we're going to fully live it, is to remember the deep. We can't leave it out of our lives without leaving the deeper part of ourselves out, too.

So how do we go deeper? Well, first we have to acknowledge there *is* a deeper, and that there is a benefit for us to connect with it. After that, it's just a matter of practice. For me, both the initial awareness *and* the practice have always come through my writing. I discovered it almost accidentally. But once you experience such depth, you never want to go back – and well, here we are.

Something Deeper is a series of written reflections, some recent and some from years ago, about everyday events that have caused me to re-discover that connection. If there *is* one, after all, and everything is part of it, then it should be evident every day, in every circumstance. And it is. We don't have to look far; we only have to look deeper.

We never know where the next profound life lesson is going to come from, and it's just as likely to come in the next five minutes as it is three days from now. The fact that it could be *any* day, shows us that they are there *every* day. Our job is to be open to receiving them. It costs us nothing but our attention.

There are 31 reflections included here, one for each day of the month. Each can be read in just a few minutes. To get the most out of them, it's best to read one each day, maybe even a few times, and limit it to that. There is also a section of written exercises, Going Deeper, in the back of the book, to encourage deeper contemplation on the daily reading. It's not necessary to do the exercise, but I would highly recommend it. There is something about writing things down that focuses our mind, and deepens any experience.

Maybe start each day with the daily reading, and end it with the written exercise. But wait until tomorrow to start the next reflection. If you run through them too quickly, you'll miss the power of them. The material world is so pervasive in our everyday reality that it takes time to begin to change our focus. But, it's time well-spent.

It doesn't require a lot of conscious thought during the day. There's nothing to study. Your contemplation will be running in the background, which will make your day better, as perceiving our deeper connection with things always does. Feel free to re-read it during the day, if it calls to you. I wrote them, and I still re-read them all the time.

It's like chipping away at the very ice that holds you up – and there is some resistance that can come with that. But once you realize that you're one with everything that lies beneath, and that you can breathe underwater just fine, it will seem completely normal to you. Once you get a glimpse of what you've been missing, you won't ever want to go back. Awe, and wonder, and gratitude seem to have that effect on us. And if you want to experience them more consistently, there's nothing left to do but to jump in.

Look at it as a grand adventure, which will begin as a journey to more deeply understand the world you live in. But in the end, the journey is an inward one, as all journeys ultimately are. It could be the journey of a lifetime. But you'll have to take it to find out.

Three-Dimensional Writing

You will notice that the reflections in this book create physical shapes, like pyramids and rectangles. I never set out to do this; the writing just evolved that way over time. I find it fun trying to fit the words into pleasant-looking shapes. It makes the process feel more playful to me. I like puzzles, and writing this way seems like I'm endlessly solving them.

"So, is it poetry, or is it prose?" people ask. "Yes," is my answer. I'm not trying to be coy. Sometimes I myself don't know what to call it. And I never really cared – until at the end of the publishing process, when we all realized how difficult it was to edit. Words, grammar, and punctuation are one thing, but when you're limited to being in a certain overall *shape*, it gets quite complex. It makes me laugh now; but there were days when we were all scratching our heads…

Which is when I began to think more deeply about it. Why *do* I write this way? And could there be a deeper meaning that I myself had not been aware of? It struck me that adding the shapes into the process was like playing 3-D chess instead of the regular game. *Yes*, I thought, it adds *depth* to everything – a deeper dimension. Oh, I know it's still two-dimensional words on a page, but *metaphorically*, it adds another dimension. Similar to the three-dimensional human design – mind, body and spirit.

But it's even more than that. Each written stanza has a rhythm to it, just as our lives do. Each is unique; no two are exactly alike – like our fingerprints, and our DNA. Each shape follows the other in an unpredictable way – just like our lives unfold. And, just like our lives, each pattern seems separate, and yet, when taken together, it all makes sense. The whole is so much greater than the sum of the parts.

Some stanzas are pure logic, many from my medical experience. Yet they are intertwined with deeper feelings from the heart, having nothing to do with that experience. Right brain and left brain work in harmony, which is how we are designed to function. Head *and* heart. We need both to be fully human. Sounds profound, and it is. But I'd be more impressed with myself if I had done it on purpose.

I realized, only after the fact, that my writing style fit perfectly with the overall theme of the book; that there are deeper things going on anywhere we care to look. And they are in play, *whether we are aware of them or not*. Oh, it was fun playing with the words, trying to fit them into all the shapes. But to see that there was a deeper, interconnected meaning to it all, which I was unknowingly participating in, was profound. There are *always* deeper things going on. May this book help you find them.

> *The mystery of life isn't a problem*
> *to solve, but a reality to experience.*
>
> FRANK HERBERT

Day 1

The Ladder of Life

Because every journey starts at home

On my 50th birthday:

What did I expect? Perfection, I suppose.
I know how unreasonable that sounds, but
when I mull things over, it's hard
to come to a different
conclusion.

I wanted my parents to be perfect.

I've always had fond memories of childhood.
Whenever I get together with my brothers and sisters,
there's always a lot of laughter as we tell all the old stories.
But looking back through adult eyes, I can now see
there were painful times, too.

Interspersed between all the laughter
were periods of anger, resentment, and isolation.
And over time, I've come to realize how growing up
in that environment has hindered me,
despite all the good times.

Even after my childhood resentments faded into forgiveness,
I've often looked back and wondered what I could have
done in life without the "holes" in my development.

If my parents had done better, how far could I have gone?
Oh, I've achieved plenty in life, but I've missed out on plenty, too.
And there are areas where I could have stepped out
confidently, but held back instead.

But as I look back with a broader perspective, I see things differently.
Having turned 50 this year, the first thing I see is that I was
raised by two people who were *half my age!*

And when I consider how much difficulty I have at 50
consistently being the person I want to be,
I gain a greater understanding.

Just what did I *expect* from two twenty-five-year-olds?
It's enough to make me laugh, as I see things now.

The prospect of those young adults, who at half my age
were presumably *twice* as clueless as I am now,
navigating their way through parenthood is
alternately comical and chilling.

I thought they *knew* how to raise children.
Didn't they take a class or something?

Certainly, there had to be some basic requirements, right?
Every parent knows there aren't, but every child assumes there are.

Yes, somehow all children expect perfect parents,
and perhaps in a perfect world, they have a right to.

Children come into the world
to be bathed in unconditional love.
Their nervous systems are wired for it.
But the world they enter is quite different
than the one they were designed for.
And sadly, no parent is
entirely whole.

Thus, by the very nature of the human experience,
every child's start in life is, on some level, less than ideal.

The fact is, our parents fought their own childhood battles,
and were wounded and scarred along the way, just like the rest of us.
Pain and emotional trauma have been around so long,
and have traveled through so many generations,
they are endemic in every family.
None are untouched.

My own pain, no matter what it is, did not originate with them,
no matter what I might have thought while growing up.
Parents are *carriers* more than originators.
Nobody grows up in a vacuum.

Just because we weren't around to witness our parents'
childhood trauma doesn't mean it wasn't there.

We're all basically in the same boat, no matter the generation.
Oh, my childhood traumas may be different from yours.
But we all come to adulthood incomplete
with something we must overcome.
Only the details are different.

And the question life puts to us is: Will we overcome it;
or will we continue to look back and wish things were different?
Or, put more directly, wish *they* had been different?

But as long as we blame our forebears,
we remain stuck in the same cycle.
Only when we let it go can
we finally move on.

Now that the veil of childhood expectation is gone,
I have a deepening love and growing compassion
for those two struggling "adults" who raised
me without a map to guide them.

They navigated by the seat of their pants, just like we all do.
Sometimes they made the right calls, and sometimes not.
But I understand now, that making the wrong ones
didn't mean they loved me any less.

However wounded, and whatever knowledge they lacked, they gave
me all they had to give, and who can ask for more than that?

Dad's gone now, with Mom perhaps not far behind.
One's time on the stage is done, and the other's nearly so,
just as I find *myself* at center stage, with the lights glaring.
"What are *you* going to do?" they seem to ask.
The question sends chills up my spine.

I'm doing the best I can, I protest,
as the glare of the lights intensifies.
I guess that's what they did.

As a child, I expected better, but I now understand
the problem was with my expectations,
and not their performance.

When I was a child, I thought like a child.
But now I see them as fellow travelers on life's journey.
They just came a little before me, and were given
the sometimes-unenviable task of
raising this little child.

And being susceptible to the same struggles
all humans are, they did it imperfectly.

I guess I always thought they were just parents.
I didn't realize until recently they were, well, *real people*.

That changes everything.

I love them more now, perhaps, than I ever have.
Maybe because I can now see through adult eyes, which
no longer hold them to impossible standards.

I thought I could be doing better now, if they'd done better then.
But I've come to believe that where they "fell short"
was the plan for me all along.

The traumas of our past are the seed of our greatest gifts.
But only after we've forgiven the traumas.
Otherwise, they just hold us back.

Looking back, I appreciate what they did more than words can say.
They took a helpless infant, and placed him on the ladder of life
as high as they could – even when he complained.
It is a gift I can never repay.

When I thought as a child, I wondered why they
didn't put me at the top of the ladder.

But now I understand: That was never their job.
I was always meant to climb the rest
of the way myself.

---

*The only time you truly become an adult,
is when you finally forgive your parents
for being just as flawed as everybody else.*

—DOUGLAS KENNEDY

Day 2

Returning Home
Because it speaks volumes

When my daughter was twelve:

My daughter asked me to watch a movie with her tonight.
She has been asking me for some time now;
and tonight, I found the time
to watch it with her.

It was a beautiful movie,
one I found extraordinarily moving.
I'm not even sure why it was so moving, honestly.
I've seen many movies, even better than this.
What was so special about this one?

I pondered it for a while, then slowly began to understand.
It wasn't the *movie*; it was her – my precious daughter.
She sought me out so we could watch it together,
wanting to spend time with Dad at an age
when many daughters don't.

She's seen the movie many times, and knows it almost by heart.
She didn't need to see it again, but wanted to – with me.
She could not have given me a
greater compliment.

As my musings expanded, I remembered my son,
who asks me to play basketball with him in the driveway.
He is taller now, and a far better player than I ever was.
If I play fairly, I never win. And I only
bend the rules for laughs.

I'm not fooling anybody.

It's never a contest, so why does he even play?
He's a confident young man, and doesn't need the ego boost
of beating his old man at a young man's game.
No, it's not about the basketball.
He plays because he wants
to spend time
with me.

There is another daughter, just finished with college.
She's finally free to go off on her own now.
Yet has chosen to come home and spend
a final summer here, with us.

But she didn't have to.
She *had* other opportunities.

And then there is the oldest child, a son.
He lives far away now, and has a life of his own.
He can come home this Christmas, and I can hear
the excitement in his voice when we talk on the phone.
Time and money are short, but he chooses
to spend both to come home.

I have always enjoyed my children.
Looking back, there weren't many moments
I didn't fully appreciate, even as they were happening.
But as they get older, to have them still want to spend
time with me, is a blessing deeper than I
could have imagined when they
were younger.

When they were small,
I thought it would last forever.
Oh, I knew in my head it wouldn't.
But my heart refused to let me believe it.
And now I'm realizing how fleeting it all really is.
Our children truly are just loaned to us for a short while.

Which is why sharing movie time with my daughter was,
for as long as I could make it last – like heaven.
A few more years, the blink of an eye,
and she, too, will be gone,
to face life on her own,
as she must.

Where did all the time go?
How could it have passed so quickly?

It's a bittersweet thing to see your children grow up
and leave the nest. There is joy in watching them grow.
And there is sadness in watching them go. But they'll always
come back; I see that now. That's what happens when you
let them go freely, despite the heartbreak of doing so.

So, fast forward twenty years – how is it going?

Better than I could have imagined.
And as you can see from all of the above,
I had imagined it pretty well.

Everyone comes back – only now with their families in tow.
Or their significant others, who also seem like part of the family.
The oldest daughter lives in Europe now,
and still comes back twice a year.
With the grandkids.

Who immediately become partners in crime
with the one who lives just down the road from us.
When they're all here together, it's quite a crowd.
And quite the chaos. But it's beautiful chaos.
And I wouldn't have it any other way.

We retell all the old stories, of course – about dirty rooms,
dented fenders, lost homework, and family vacations.
But there's much more now. More to laugh about.
More to share. More stories to tell.
More of everything.

Twenty years ago,
I foresaw it being great.
But it turned out even better.

What's the secret, you ask?

Well, I do remember thinking when they were little,
no matter what the stage of childhood,
that there was a tiny adult lying
somewhere inside – dormant,
but ever watchful.

And I always tried to respect that unseen adult,
even when it was housed in a somewhat unruly child.
And now that they're grown, I'm so glad I did.
It has allowed us to become friends now.
And there's nothing better than
being friends with your
adult children.

Every event in the life of a family is like a thread.
And over the years, they're woven into a beautiful tapestry,
one that only they share, and that becomes more
beautiful with each passing year.

And as I consider the yet-to-be-finished tapestry of *this* family,
I am content; and I realize that I have accomplished much in life.
Because a man whose grown children come home
when they no longer have to is a success,
no matter what else he has done.

To see them smile when they walk in the door,
and brush away a tear when they leave, speaks volumes.
Volumes, which are written with their hearts, not their words.

And what do those volumes say?

That they feel safe here. That they feel welcome.
That they don't feel judged, but are instead celebrated.
That it's okay to be who they are. That there are no expectations.
It means that the nest was warm enough back in the day,
and there are enough sweet memories, that they
look forward to returning to it when they can.
And, even more meaningful, that they
want to share that experience
with their own kids.

To know that, in partnership with my wife,
I have created such a space for them,
gives me a deeper satisfaction
than I know how to
describe.

And my only job now,
is to be at peace.
And enjoy.

---

*Hanging out with your adult children
is like visiting the most beautiful
and precious parts of your life.*

—UNKNOWN

Day 3

A Long and Winding Road

Because it's never too late to see things differently

"I'll *forgive*, but I won't *forget!*" the angry man said,
about a person and an event that time has
long since clouded over in my mind.

I only remember I was a mere observer, and not
the subject of his ire – at least not that time,
there usually being plenty of it
to go around.

Funny, I can no longer remember
what caused those words, but I remember
the words like it was yesterday.

Yeah, right! I thought to myself at the time; *Get back to me on that.*
Of course, he hadn't forgiven, and likely hasn't to this day.

I remember the words exactly as he spoke them.
But a more honest translation would
go something like this:

"I'll never forget what you did.
And I'll hate you for it until the day I die."

It was hard not to laugh at the grand declaration
of forgiveness, despite the obvious lack of it.

But I kept my laughter in check,
given the heated nature of
the discussion.

It was a partners' meeting, as I recall,
which all seemed to be heated back in the day,
for reasons I'm still trying
to figure out.

It's interesting, though, that after all these years,
I would remember those few words
more than any of the rest of it.

And I got to wondering,
why *do* I remember those words,
when everything else is lost to history?
Could it be that I, myself, have not forgiven?

Oh, I don't mean about this. I just found this scenario amusing.
But I wasn't the one in his crosshairs, at least not this time,
though there were plenty of times I was.
Yes, there were plenty of
times for us all.

And if this scenario feels a bit heavy, even after all this time,
could it be a sign that I myself have not let things go?

Or was I judging a clearly wounded man, who happened
to find himself at the top of an organization he
was not emotionally suited to lead?

They were interesting questions, I had to admit,
as I began to feel less certain about
the whole thing.

Wait a minute, what's this? I asked myself,
as a scene began to slowly unfold in my head.

It was a little boy, a five-year old, I think.
And he was trembling – so upset he couldn't move,
so terrified he couldn't even cry.

There was a large figure towering over him,
possibly his father, saying things I couldn't quite hear.
The figure was clearly berating the boy mercilessly.

Berating him for what?
For some transgression, no doubt.
But I don't think the "what" really mattered.
I'm sure I was seeing just a small glimpse
of what was a recurring pattern.

It seemed so unfair.
I don't care what the boy did.
He didn't deserve *that* kind of treatment.

No child does.

I felt a mixture of sadness and anger;
sadness for the helpless child,
and anger at the adult,

who was clearly
bullying him.

And yet, I was powerless to do anything about it,
since I was witnessing an event from a long-distant past.
The scene began to fade, but the tears remained on my cheeks.

Imagine that, I thought to myself sadly.
The boy was so frightened he couldn't even cry.

I found myself hoping in some magical way that the tears
I was experiencing would help heal him. But I had no idea how.

The scene disappeared, I came back to the present;
and suddenly, I didn't find the original
"I'll forgive, but I won't forget,"
quite so comical
any more.

Understanding the trembling five-year old inside the adult
had given me reason to pause, and reconsider
my attitude toward him.

It doesn't make anything he did less damaging.
But it does make it more understandable.
And more importantly, it took the
emotional charge out of
everything.

OK, I did lose the amusement of this particular incident.
But the sting was also gone from all those times

when I *had* found myself in his crosshairs,
which is a pretty good tradeoff.

On top of that, other memories started coming back,
of times when he wasn't so angry, times he had helped me,
and had gone out of his way to show kindness.

They're nice memories. They make me smile.
But they'd been lost to me all this time,
covered over by a single
negative one.

Carrying a grudge is a double-edged sword, it seems;
only both edges of the sword are harmful to us.
Not only do we have to bear the ongoing
weight of the troubling memory,
but we also lose sight of
the good things.

Now that I can look back and smile,
I can see it's just not worth it.

Maybe our troubling memories are an invitation.
Maybe this story stayed in my head for so long for a reason,
when thousands of other interactions from the same
time period had been lost to my memory.

Well, if so, I'm grateful.

And happy that our souls have a way of tapping us
on the shoulder, ever so gently, and letting us know that

we have some internal work to do if we're
going to stay emotionally healthy.

The road to compassion, it seems, can be a long one.
But it's a road worth taking, no matter
how long it takes to find it.

---

*Let our hearts be stretched out in compassion
toward others, for everyone is walking
his or her own difficult path.*

—DIETER D. UCHTDORF

Day 4

The Last Drop

Because now is all we have

The last drop of wine hung there for what seemed like forever.
As the waiter held the bottle over my glass, the drop
seemingly did *not* want to fall into it.
And for a few moments,
time stood still.

We were at a restaurant in New York City,
about twenty years ago. Just my wife and I.

I don't remember the name of the restaurant,
what we had for dinner, or even what
the waiter looked like.

I just remember that he seemed like a nice young man,
personable, and yet professional, at the same time.
I've seen a lot of waiters pour wine in my day.
But I've never seen anyone do what he did.

As the last drop of wine hung precariously
from the bottle – he did nothing.
He watched. And he waited.
And that was all.

Would it finally fall off into my glass?
Would he wipe it away with his cloth?

Or would he get tired of waiting,
pull the bottle away, and
let the last drop fall
where it may?

It's hard for me to believe I was
spellbound over all this, but I was.

How long did he wait?
Hard to say – ten seconds, maybe?
But it seemed like
an eternity.

What kind of focus did that take, I wondered?
Surely, he had lots of other stuff to do.
Waiters are always trying to do
three things at once,
aren't they?

But judging by how focused he was, you would have
thought this was his only job of the evening.

He was intensely present, my wife and I decided,
as we discussed the whole thing later.
It affected both of us deeply.

I was mesmerized by that drop of wine.
And I haven't forgotten it to this day.

I could understand if I were watching a
master surgeon at work, or perhaps
a world-famous artist paint.

But a waiter pouring a glass of wine?

It's just a reminder that intense presence is powerful.
And that anybody can change the atmosphere around them,
no matter what their job or walk of life,
simply by intensely focusing on
whatever they're doing
in the moment.

To be fully focused in the present moment,
is to bring magic into that moment.
And everyone around you is
positively impacted.

In church, we sometimes hear about the "presence of God."
It's a palpable sense of immense power that happens occasionally.
But what are we feeling, really? It can't be *God's* presence.
Isn't God *always* present – by definition?

No, they're talking about their *own* presence.
And the intensity of having so many people
in the same place with hearts open,
and in a state of gratitude,
focusing on the
same thing.

They're in *resonance* with each other. It's palpable. *And* powerful.
Magical things happen in that atmosphere – even miraculous things.
It's something you'll never experience at the supermarket.

But individually, we can bring the same power into
any moment, by fully focusing on whatever we're doing,
and not fretting over yesterday, or worrying about tomorrow.

In the midst of any task, if we find ourselves wondering
in the background what we're having for lunch, or if our team
won last night, or how our investments are doing,
then we're not fully present; because each
one of these diminishes our focus,
and thereby, the power that
we bring into the
moment.

By definition, life only happens in the present moment.
Which means that, if our minds are fragmented and
our attention is scattered, we're not fully living.

And in *that* moment twenty years ago, thanks to our waiter,
the three of us *were* living. It was magical,
memorable, and impactful,
all at the same time.

I think about the waiter, from time to time.
Where is he now? What has his life been like?
After some thought, I decide he's had a wonderful life.

Because you don't pay attention to the last drop of wine,
without giving the same care to the other
details of your life as well.

An excellent life comes from paying attention to the "small things,"
or better said, without considering *anything* a small thing.
Because everything deserves our full attention.

What's the message of "the last drop of wine?"
That there are deep life lessons to be found in places
we'd least expect, which is why it's good
to always be paying attention.

Miracles occur all day, every day,
but we have to be able to perceive them.
When we are fully in the moment, we will resonate
with the miracles that are trying to reach us,
which will cause us to attract them.

And the best way to make sure we're fully present
is to catch ourselves when our minds start to
wander off into the past or the future,
both being mental constructs,
neither having any
life in them.

No, life is here and now, and that's
the only place we're ever going to find it.

Curiosity is now. Wonder is now. Joy is now.
Gratitude is now. And Love is now.
And maybe *now*, we've gotten
down to the real point.

Live in the moment, as much as you can.
And use curiosity, wonder, joy, gratitude, and love
as your tools to measure whether you're there or not.
When you feel them, then you're there.
When they're absent, so are you.

Good luck in your quest.
It will take you to some beautiful places;
or rather, it will cause you to recognize
the beautiful places that are
already there.

---

*Realize deeply that the present
moment is all you will ever have.*

—ECKHART TOLLE

Day 5

A Peaceful Evening

Because everything is a miracle, if we just stop long enough to notice

I went for a bike ride this evening, as I often do.
And for some reason I decided to stop
and sit by the lake for a while.

I ride by there often, and I always
appreciate the scenery, but have never
stopped before to just sit.

It's not a big lake,
just one of those man-made things,
quite common in golf course communities.
Oh, I don't play golf. I just live here
for the natural beauty.
And for evenings
like these.

And *this* evening, for some reason,
I found this particular spot intriguing.

It was a beautiful evening,
cool, with a soft breeze.

The sunlight fell gently across my shoulders,
as it does when the day starts to fade,
and the world becomes calm.

It reminded me of the beautiful autumn days of
childhood, when just being outdoors
brought me a sense of peace.

I looked up at the clouds and laughed,
as I saw animals, boats, and dozens of other
oddities that morphed into other
shapes almost as quickly
as they had appeared.

Surely, these were different shapes
than the ones I saw as a child.
And yet they looked
so familiar.

Could they be the same, I wondered?
Do clouds experience time?
It's the same water vapor.
So, who's to say?

So many years ago,
and yet, it feels like the same:
the breeze, the fading sunlight, all of it.

A few birds flew overhead.
Why do the two small birds follow
the larger one so closely,

imitating its every
move?

They're not the same type of bird.
They don't look like they're hunting.
And they're not fighting.
Are they playing?
Do birds play?

There are no real answers, of course.
And I wasn't looking for any.

They were more about a sense of wonder, I suppose.
And gratitude, for whatever it is that weaves
this beautiful tapestry, and allows me to
take part in it – when I slow down
enough to notice, that is.

The sound of a plane pierced the quiet,
having just taken off from the airport nearby.
And my gaze followed it as it ascended into the
evening sky, disappearing into the clouds.

Who's on that plane? I wondered.
Are they happy? Sad? Healthy? Sick?
Where are they going? And why?

There I go again with all the questions, I thought to myself.
But I couldn't stop asking them. Nor did I want to.

Questions are beautiful, I've come to understand.
Perhaps especially when they don't demand an answer,
but simply allow us to let the wonder in.

All the times I've ridden by there …
Why haven't I stopped before?

Why do I remember the times I did this as a child
as if they were a mere five minutes ago?
I'd swear they're the same clouds.
Could time be less linear
than we thought?

And much more mysterious?

It was getting late, and the sunlight was fading;
time to head home and get back to my life.
Or was I leaving life to go
back to the noise?

Hmmm … I'll have to contemplate that one, I thought.
And I promised myself I'd return there from time to time,
though I wondered whether it was the "there" that was special,
or if it was more about the state of my soul;
and perhaps I could find this *anywhere*.

Just as the child did so long ago,
in a place so very far away,
yet now seems so near.

Yes, it's all a wonder.
And, perhaps our purpose in life,
is just to notice …

The important thing is not to stop questioning. Curiosity has its own reason for existing. One cannot help but be in awe when one contemplates the mysteries of eternity, of life, of the marvelous structure of reality.

—ALBERT EINSTEIN

Day 6

A Mundane Day
Because there's no such thing

So, how do I make today a meaningful day, I wondered?
Mostly to myself, I suppose, since no one was around to hear me.

I don't plan on going anywhere, have nothing on the agenda,
and won't be interacting with anyone that I know of.
I could organize a few things, I suppose,
maybe take care of some things
around the house.

But all in all, it seems like a pretty mundane day.
So, what does it matter, then? I mean, what's the point?
If I am to make every day count, what about days like today,
when I won't be on anyone's stage, and thus unable
to impact anyone in a positive way?

How do you know?

It was an unexpected voice, from out of nowhere.
Oh, it wasn't audible. I can't say I actually "heard" it.
But I did *hear* it. And it was pretty clear.

And I *had* just asked a question, of sorts.
So, I decided to bypass the chaotic thoughts
racing through my head, wondering

where the voice came from,
and just listen.

It turned out to be one of my better decisions.
Because the unknown voice continued ...

You don't know that you won't have a chance to impact anyone.
That's just how things look to your logical mind.

You're writing this, first of all,
*and you never know where **that** will go.*
*And just because there's no **outlook***
for meaningful interactions,
doesn't mean there
won't be any.

Be sure as you approach any given day
that you leave room in your mind for the unexpected.
When you do, life will seem like the adventure it really is,
which makes it clear that it's your outlook that's
the problem, and not the coming day.

Mundane days are a figment of your imagination.
They do not occur in nature. You create them in your mind,
believe your own mental construct, and then spend
a perfectly good day as if it doesn't matter.

*But **every** day matters, in ways both great and small.*
Where you go wrong is when you try to define which is which.

*The truth is, there **are** no mundane days.*
"Mundane" exists only in your head.

Not talking to anyone today, or so you think?
Not doing anything today, or so you think?

It doesn't matter.

You'll be thinking today.
You'll be considering the future, and the past.
You'll be mulling over situations in your life, and in the world.
*You may not **physically** interact with the "outside world,"*
*but make no mistake, you **will** be*
interacting with it.

And it's best to make those mental interactions meaningful and positive.
The thoughts and feelings you hold for others are prayers of a sort.
Never forget this, and it will guide you to a meaningful life.
You can accomplish much sitting home
not speaking to anyone at all.

Anytime you hold positive thoughts in your heart for a loved one,
or imagine a positive outcome to a situation, it is meaningful.
Anytime you hold compassionate or forgiving thoughts
for an adversary, you are accomplishing something.
Anytime you imagine a more peaceful future,
anytime you are grateful, it is meaningful.

Focus on these, and every day will seem
like the grand adventure it truly is.

*There is magic everywhere around you, in every moment of every day.
There are deep life lessons available to you in the simplest of things;
the only question being, are you able to recognize them?*

*Every day is completely unpredictable from a human perspective.
When you label anything mundane, much less an entire day,
you only show that you are missing the point.*

*But no matter – life is an endless stream of mysteries, adventures,
and profound moments that can touch your heart.
And since it **is** an endless stream, it doesn't
matter when you decide
to jump in.*

*At the very least, remember that every positive thought
you have helps heal both yourself and the world.*

*And every negative thought serves to degrade the same.
Which means – everything you do matters,
even when outwardly, it looks like
you're doing nothing at all.*

*So, as you can see, not only are there no mundane days,
but also, no mundane tasks, and no mundane moments.*

*And if you can be fully present for each and every one of those moments,
and in everything you do, you will lead a life of meaning and purpose.*

You owe this to yourself, as well as to the world, no?

*When the word "mundane" comes to mind, remember it's not real,
remind yourself to look a little deeper – and when you do,
a world of wonder will open up to you.
It's been there all along, of course.
It's just been waiting for
you to notice.*

Wow, that was more than I bargained for!
After sitting with it for a while, I decided it was, indeed,
deep wisdom, and I should take it to heart. So, I did.
And nothing has ever been the same.

---

*The world is full of magic things, patiently
waiting for our senses to grow sharper.*

—W. B. YEATS

Day 7

The Placebo Effect

Because, sometimes, the hardest thing to see is what's right in front of us

I recently joined an Intention Group, just out of curiosity. It's like a secular prayer group, where we meet and spend time focusing our positive intention on helping each other create something in our life, typically health or business-related.

I have to say, the results so far have been pretty amazing. Besides my own personal manifestations, it has been a joy to watch others benefit from my time and attention.

There is a fairly large network of Intention Groups. And there's a lot of talk in them about spontaneous healings, meaning healings, from even serious diseases, without a known medical cause.

And *apparently*, they're more common than I thought. I've heard about spontaneous healings before, though I've never seen any personally; probably a side effect of spending too much time in hospitals.

But now that I'm running in different circles,
I'm starting to hear about them a lot more.

It's a fascinating subject, one that touches on
the depth of who we are as humans
and the powers we've been
endowed with.

We know if you give someone a sugar pill
and tell them it's real, they can heal all on their own.
They call it the placebo effect, for lack of a better term, probably.
From a medical perspective, it's a code word for trickery,
a nuisance that gets in the way of drug research,
and nothing more than that.

But *why* do people get better, if there's no medicine in the pill?
It's a simple question; but it's one the medical system doesn't ask,
possibly because the system is so complex,
and the question so simple.

It would seem that their own belief
they'd get better, actually made them so.
I don't see another logical answer,
hard as I might look for one.

"It's all in their head!"
said a voice, from out of nowhere.
It was one of my old medical school professors,
sounding as crotchety in my imagination
as he did back in the day.

I didn't challenge my professors much back then.
But buoyed by the passing years and
a lifetime of experience,
I felt a lot bolder.

What do you mean, it's all in their head?
I pushed back. *They're better, aren't they?*

"It's all in their head!"
he said again, dismissively,
with an arrogance that brought back
distasteful memories from a now-distant past.

So, what if it's only in their head?
I pushed back. *Better is better, isn't it?*
*And last time I checked, the head **is** actually*
part of the body, so how does that not count?
Besides, you're dead and gone, now, which means
you're only in my head, too. So, should I disregard what
you taught me because you're less tangible now,
or use what's only "in my head"
as a valuable tool?

He didn't answer, so I went on.

Despite your outdated views, I think I will keep you around,
I said, as I softened a bit, realizing he had been born
not in the *last* century, but the one before *that*.

He was only doing the best he could with the information
available to him at the time – kind of like we all do.

I am appreciative of all you taught me, I continued.
*But it will have to be modified, due to the passage of time,
and the inexorable onward march of new information.
You'd expect no less from me if you were really here.*

Oh, the information itself is not new.
It's just a new way of looking at *old* information.
But it's revolutionary, just the same,
since a new way of looking at
life results in – a new life.

And as part of my new life, I think I'll send a posse to rescue
poor Placebo, who, last I checked, was chained up
in the basement of the Drug Factory, relegated
to the quality control line, using only
a *fraction* of his talents.

People will be outraged, years from now, when they realize
that Placebo had been hidden away from public view all this time,
by a medical system that's supposed to be about healing,
but is sometimes about so many other things.

"What!?" they'll exclaim.
*"That's like Einstein being stuck
working in the patent office because
he couldn't find a 'real' physics job."*

Yes, someday, we won't need to trick people
into using the power of their mind for healing,
and the sugar pill will be a thing of the past.

The healing power of the human mind will then
be common knowledge. And the "miraculous healings"
we talk about now, will cease to be so miraculous,
since they will actually have a cause, albeit
a mental, rather than a physical, one.

And once people realize they can experience relief from
physical maladies by mental focus and positive intention alone,
they'll realize what *else* they can accomplish.
Yes, *maybe*, we'll realize that the power
to heal the world lies within
our own hearts
and minds.

And *that* will be a wonderful day for us all.

---

*The best medicine we have
is the power of our own minds.*

—LYNNE MCTAGGART

Day 8

A Boy and His Dog

Because you never forget

A friend's dog passed away last week; and, knowing
how difficult that can be, my heart hurts for her.

Sure, some would say it's just a dog.
But considering how deep the bond can be,
there's no "just" about it. It's a loss,
and a deep one at that.

People are always trying to quantify love, thinking love
for a human means more than for a dog, which
is presumably slightly more than for a cat,
and, I guess, a lot more than
for a turtle.

And while on a certain level, this may be true,
it's just as true that we never really love anything.
Rather, we *are* love, in our deepest essence, and the things
we "love" cause us to connect with the love that's already within us.
In other words, they help us connect with who we really are.

When I think of my friend's loss,
memories come flooding back of my own dog,
who, herself, has long since passed away.

I've had other dogs in my life.
And though I fondly remember them all,
there's only one who *changed* my life.

She was my first dog.
And my best dog.

I don't think about her much anymore.
But the passing of my friend's dog reminded me
of how special our bond was; and I realize,
that even after all this time,
I still miss her.

It sounds funny to hear myself say that,
since she passed away nearly half a century ago.
Almost in a different lifetime, it now seems.

The boy who loved her no longer even exists,
at least on the outside; though what I feel in my heart
when I think about her tells me he's still
alive and well on the inside.

I've had a full life, by any standards:
attended medical school, authored a book,
climbed mountains, traveled the world.

And, more importantly, created a beautiful family
that continues to expand, and yet seems to
grow closer with each passing year.

So why, then, do I still feel emotional
over a dog who died nearly a lifetime ago?

She was special to the whole family, not just to me.
She went to the beach with us, played softball with us,
and went pretty much everywhere we did,
mostly without the need of a leash.

But for me, the deeper things were what mattered.

She was the emotional glue in a family that
had difficulty showing emotion,
the one I went to for hugs
in a family where there
were no hugs.

Oh, I know, dogs can't hug, technically.
But in my mind, she hugged me every time she laid
next to me on the floor, or hopped on the couch with me,
or into bed, whenever Mom would allow it.

And it was okay for me to lay my head on her
and listen to her heartbeat. Yes, she loved that.

No, she wasn't human; but looking back,
she filled a vital space for a sensitive little boy
who didn't know there was a space that needed filling.

How close were the two of us?

When I was little, there was a time when I was very ill.
Oh, it wasn't life-threatening, but I was sick enough
that my mom still talked about it years later,
though I have almost no memory of it.

I only know that I had to stay in a darkened room for days,
and Mom felt sorry for me; so, she let the dog sleep in my bed,
something which was otherwise strictly forbidden.
I only vaguely remember the darkened room,
and have no memory at all of feeling bad.
But *do* remember how special I
felt that she got to sleep
in the bed with me.

She was the family dog, to be sure, and everyone loved her.
But I always felt that she and I had a special bond,
that I was the only one who really *saw* her,
who looked deeply into her eyes
and actually *knew* her.

And even more than that, now that I look back,
I realize that *she knew me,* likely better than I knew myself.
I didn't know how to describe it at the time,
but I felt *alive* when I was with her.

It may have been the first stirrings of my soul's awakening.
I didn't know what it was. I only knew how it felt.
And that I never wanted it to end.

She used to go with me on my paper route when I was older.
It was quite a hike to get there, and it was an apartment complex,
so there were lots of stairs to go up and down.
And she would climb every one
of them with me.

But she was older then, as well.
And I could hear her whimper in pain
as she clumsily tried to navigate the stairs
because her joints hurt so much.

I felt bad for her, so I started making her stay
at the bottom of the stairs until I came back down.
And then, finally, I had to make her stay home.

It breaks my heart to think
of how much pain she was in.
And how willing she was to endure it.

Just to be with me.

As far as I was concerned, we'd had her all my life,
since I have no early memories that don't include her.

Part of me thought she'd be around forever.
But, of course, she grew old, was in too much pain,
and my parents had her put to sleep.

The hardest thing was,
I never got to say goodbye.

I was in the middle of a
high school wrestling tournament.
And they were worried it might upset me.
So, they took her to the vet and had
her put down without
telling me.

One day she was there – and the next she wasn't.
It was left for me to ask, "Where's Lady?"

I'm still not sure why I had to ask.

But I never mentioned it to them.
Parenting is a tough job, and you have to
make a lot of judgment calls, not all of which
turn out to be the right ones.
And this one wasn't.

How could they possibly think high school wrestling
was more important than saying goodbye
to my lifelong companion?

No, it was the wrong call, and I thought so at the time,
though I didn't realize until now how much
not saying goodbye mattered to me.
I never really cried over her.
Until now.

I've thought about her over the years, from time to time.
But didn't realize until now, that I never really grieved her loss;

not until my friend mentioned her own dog,
and how much she had meant to her.

Then it all came flooding back, as if it were yesterday.
Maybe that's how we know love is eternal;
because it's never really gone,
even though the object of
our affection may be.

It can lay dormant in our souls for decades, undisturbed,
and suddenly feel as alive as our own breath.

I can almost feel her curly, black, bear-like fur.
And see how she looked at me with
those deep brown eyes,
admiring me.

Just for being me.

Grieving is a necessary part of the human condition.
It's our soul's way of adjusting to loss, to a new normal.
It can be postponed, even for decades,
but if we are to truly be whole,
we have to go through it.

Grief is a bridge we must cross, to leave behind a past
that no longer exists, and enter a future which
is built on the very foundation we
now have to leave behind.

If we avoid the bridge, we will still have the memories.
But if we're willing to brave it, the memories will
be more beautiful, and more cherished than
they would have been otherwise.

Crossing the bridge allows our grief to work its magic.
Yes, it's painful. But the pain is temporary.
The benefit lasts for the
rest of our lives.

I'm sorry for my friend's loss, and for her pain.
But I'm grateful she shared both with me.
My life is richer for it, as it put me in
touch with long-buried pain
of my own that I had
never processed.

How fortunate that little boy was.
And he didn't even know it.

Such a bond is powerfully healing, no matter what form it takes.
And I'm grateful to a Universe that sends us such things,
in unexpected ways, and in unexpected places,
filling gaps in our lives we didn't
even know were there.

---

*Until one has loved an animal, a part of
one's soul remains unawakened.*

—ANATOLE FRANCE

Day 9

Grateful

Because it always pays to ask

I was taking out the trash this evening.
And as I approached the curb, I saw my neighbor
as she passed by my house, walking her dog.
"How are you doing?" I asked.

"I'm *grateful*," she replied, with a forcefulness that surprised me.
She walks by my house often, so there are a lot of cursory greetings,
and her dog and I have become buddies of a sort.
But this was the first time she'd said *that!*

Grateful for what? was the logical question, but I never asked it.
Yes, I was a bit curious, but I quickly decided that
the "what" didn't really matter.

It was the lightness of her step, the smile on her face,
and her overall positive energy that struck me.
I see her all the time, but this evening,
she seemed different somehow.

She was just so ... happy, I remember thinking.
So, I left her statement alone, not seeking further detail.

And, though I'm still somewhat curious, I am reminded that
whatever it was that made her so grateful isn't nearly
as important as the fact that she *was* grateful.

Yes, it's the gratitude itself that carries the magic.
The reason for it is just the vehicle we take to get there.
The reasons are interchangeable, and ultimately unimportant.
It's the state of mind that's important, and of the heart,
since gratitude is always a combination of both.

I'm sure my neighbor has
had many happy walks with her dog.
And, while I don't know about the others,
I can guarantee this was
one of them.

And not because of her statement, but because I could *feel* it.
The joy and positivity she felt shone like a beacon.
She didn't need a flashlight that evening.
Because she *was* the light.

I've come to believe the formula for a happy life is simple:
Whatever you think, say, or do, that causes you
to feel gratitude in any form,
do more of that.

And whatever you think, say, or do that
causes you to feel less grateful,
do less of that.

That's it. Nothing else.
The rest is just details, anyway.

I didn't stop and chat with my neighbor that night.
But, in a deeper sense, we had a beautiful conversation.

Just not a conventional one.

Such is the nature of gratitude.
It doesn't just make us more aware
of the miracles around us.
It *creates* them.

And considering its positive impact on our
physical, mental, and spiritual state,
gratitude itself is a miracle.

One with the power to change a simple walk with your dog
into something deeper and more far-reaching,
affecting those around you more than
you might ever know …

---

*It is not joy that makes us grateful;
it is gratitude that makes us joyful.*

—DAVID STEINDL-RAST

Day 10

The Pizza Guy

Because we all get hungry

I was watching TV the other evening, and
as it sometimes happens, I suddenly
realized that I was hungry.

Why?
I don't know.
It's anybody's guess;
though maybe it had to do with
the pizza commercial I had just seen.

But regardless, I did what I so often do in those situations,
I called the pizza delivery guy, and ordered a pizza.
"Thirty minutes," he said. "Thanks for ordering."
"Sure," I replied, then hung up the phone,
and went back to the TV.

It's a ritual that's been repeated countless times,
in my home, and in others across the country.

The thirty minutes passed uneventfully,
the doorbell rang, and there he was, right on time.
After a brief greeting, he handed me the pizza; I gave him a tip.
Then he was on his way to the next delivery.
And I was on my way to dinner.

There was nothing at all remarkable about the whole thing.
Except for some reason, this evening, I considered
what *didn't* happen during the
thirty-minute wait.

Mostly, that I never doubted he would come.
In fact, the possibility never even occurred to me.
I guess because he *always* comes.

Oh, I can remember a time or two he didn't show up
and I had to call again; irritating to be sure, but it's a rare event.
In fact, I can't remember the last time it happened.
And once in a while he's late,
but not often enough
to worry about.

No, I gave neither of those possibilities a second thought
while I watched TV in perfect peace, knowing
that what I had put into motion with
my phone call was a done deal.
I had asked, and trusted it
would be done.

It dawned on me, though, that despite the
everyday nature of pizza delivery,
there might be some lessons
to be learned.

I thought about how
once I ordered my pizza,
I had complete faith it would arrive.

I didn't worry. I didn't fret. I didn't doubt.
And thus, remained in perfect peace during my wait.

In fact, sometimes, if I'm not too hungry,
I'm *so* much at peace I almost forget I called.

How can I have so much peace?
Because I have an unshakable belief,
without an ounce of doubt, that he'll show up,
just like he said he would.

Then I thought about my prayer requests,
and how different I am with them.

I'm told I have not because I ask not, so I ask.
And am also told, that if I ask, and don't doubt,
but instead believe I already have it, then it's done;
the transaction is sealed, and the only thing missing is time.

Which is where things begin to break down.
Because rarely am I as much at peace after my prayers
as I am waiting for the pizza I just ordered.
I wish I could report otherwise.
I just can't.

Here's how it usually goes:

I ask, feel good about asking,
and feel good about the entire process.
Until about ten minutes later, when I'm back

in my material reality, which is when the fun begins.
And I begin wondering if God heard me;
or maybe I'm not worthy in some way.
Maybe I ran a red light last week,
or was rude to the waitress,
or, who knows?

Maybe He answers prayers for saints, but not for normal people.
Or maybe the whole prayer thing is made up;
or, God forbid, he doesn't even exist.
(Isn't that an oxymoron?)

And why am I talking to somebody I can't even see?
Can I *really* know if somebody's listening?
Or if there's even anybody there?

I'm not saying these things run through my *conscious* mind.
But I'm pretty sure they run through my subconscious,
judging by the angst and doubt I sometimes
feel over things I've asked for.

I think it's pretty normal, actually. At least I hope it is.
I mean, if faith were that easy, *everybody* would be a saint,
which they most definitely are not.

Yes, I'm convinced
that to one extent or another,
we all struggle to have faith in something
we cannot see with our own eyes.

We *say* that we believe in God.
And that we know God answers prayers.
But on some level, part of us is not quite sure,
the "not quite sure" part being minimal on good days,
and much larger than that on the bad ones.

We're all a mixture of belief and unbelief.
It's part of the human dilemma.

Sounds reasonable enough.
But what brings it into perspective,
is imagining the pizza delivery scenario
as though it were part of
my spiritual life.

And this is how it might go:

I pick up the phone, dial a few numbers,
and hear a voice on the other end. It's a real voice,
at least it sounds like one; but I never see
who I'm actually talking to.

An agreement is made concerning the pizza, and then I wait.
But what if he doesn't come? He said he would,
but how can I really know?

There are a thousand things that could happen.
He could forget. The driver might not find my house.
They could be out of pizza sauce; or even worse, pepperoni.

I try to watch TV, but I can't concentrate
for all the worry about the pizza.

If I wait the thirty minutes, and he doesn't show, *then* what?
I'll be even hungrier, and I'll have to start all over again.

Would I even call the same guy back?
Why? When he's already let me down once?
No, if it didn't work the first time, there's
no reason to think it would the next.

So, I decided if things don't work out, I'll call somebody else.
I know my thirty-minute wait started five minutes ago,
but one has to plan for all contingencies.

I turn off the TV, because I just can't concentrate.
And come to think of it, the show wasn't that great anyway.

And I'm *hungry*.

Maybe it would have been better to just pick up the pizza.
I know it takes more time, but I wouldn't have to deal with all *this*.

I'm beginning to think faith is overrated, anyway.
Jesus talked about all the things we could do
if we just had the faith of a mustard seed.
But what does that even mean?
Do they put mustard
seeds on pizza?

It's been twenty minutes, and still nothing.
I know he's not due for another ten minutes yet,
but I'm getting pretty antsy about it.
And the whole process is
beginning to feel
like a hassle.

In fact, though I order it all the time,
I'm not sure how much I even *like* pizza.

Twenty-five minutes, and he's *still* not here.
He's not going to come; I can feel it.

It makes me angry.
I've even paid him already.
I know I could get my money back
from the credit card company.
But we all know how much
of a hassle *that* is.

Thirty minutes, the doorbell rings; it's the pizza guy, as promised.
After a brief greeting, he hands me the pizza, I give him a tip.
Then he's on his way to the next delivery.
And I'm on my way to dinner.

The problem is, I'm so mentally exhausted
that I'm not even hungry anymore.
I no longer have the energy.

I put the pizza in the fridge, turn in early,
and on my way to bed, I have an alarming thought:
What if I had to actually *pray* for my pizza?

Now, *that* might be a problem.

Faith is like a blind man looking in a black room for a black cat, that isn't there; and finding it.

—OSCAR WILDE

Day 11

An Old Friend

Because they're timeless

An old friend called today.
He had been thinking about me,
and decided to reach out.

We were best friends in high school
and for a while afterwards,
before he moved away
and we lost touch.

How long has it been since we've talked?
I'm not sure exactly – decades, I guess;
longer than I want to say.

There had never been a falling out.
Normal life happened to us both, I suppose,
in different ways, on different coasts,
meeting different people,
having different
experiences.

Did we just grow apart? I wouldn't put it that way.
We just lost touch, as people sometimes do.
It never seemed like a bad thing.
It wasn't anybody's fault.

Everything is only
for a season.

Yet, when we talked today, it was like no time had passed.
It sounds odd to say that after all these years;
I mean, how can that even be?

We were friends for just a few short years,
and have lived nearly a lifetime since then.

Considering that we're nearer the end of life than the beginning,
and how early in life our friendship was, it represents
only the tiniest fraction of our mutual experience.
Yet, I've spent most of today remembering
how close a friend he was, and
just how meaningful the
relationship was.

It was much more meaningful than I'd realized at the time.
And more meaningful than linear time would suggest it should be.
With the obvious lesson being that soul connections
cannot be measured in linear time.
They're deeper than that.
And more enduring.

It was interesting to hear about his life and his career.
But I didn't press him for details, as he didn't press me for any.
I know he's had joys and heartaches
we didn't have time to go into,
just as I have.

Funny, I would have thought catching up
on lifetimes spent separately would have focused
more on the details; but the details
didn't seem to matter.

What mattered was, despite the decades
and the completely separate life trajectories,
it felt just like our old high school conversations;
about girls, and football, and whatever else we thought
was important, back in the day – when life was a lot simpler.
I don't even remember now what else we used to talk about.
But it doesn't really matter; and probably never did.

I'm glad he called. I've been celebrating it all day.
It's like recapturing a small, but important piece of my life.
I've always had fond memories of our friendship.
But over the years, it had become like an old
black and white picture on the wall.
It's something I know happened,
but now seemed so distant,
I had forgotten the
richness of it.

The memory was nice, but it no longer moved me.
But today, in that brief time of reconnecting,
everything came flooding back.

I can't say I remember things differently now,
but the memories have a new life to them.
They feel fresh again, as if decades

of rust was brushed away
in the space of a single
phone call.

And I'm reminded just how good a friend he was.
And how much I missed him when he left.
But I see now, he was never really gone.
Deep friendships may hibernate,
even for nearly a lifetime.
But they never die.
I see that now.

So, thank you, my friend,
For reaching out after all this time,
and reminding me how fleeting life is.
And how precious those souls are
with whom we have shared
an important part of it,
no matter how
briefly.

Yes, we are all just passing through,
which is good to contemplate
from time to time.

It keeps us from taking things for granted,
not least of which are the friends
we've made along the way.

We'll have to let go of all our material things at the end,
since those are tied to the realm of space and time.

But since friendships aren't defined by space and time,
is it possible we get to keep those connections
wherever we're headed next?
I'd like to think so.

I know I plan on appreciating them more while I'm here.
And I know my friend feels the same way.
Oh, he didn't say it in words.
But I know that's what
he meant.

Because to friends, the words don't matter.
And I see now, that they never did.

---

*Old friends never get old. Whenever they meet,
time rolls back, and they become young again.*

—SYED BADIUZZAMAN

Day 12

Dare to Dream

Because we're capable of so much more than we believe

Recently, a friend completed an Ironman Triathlon.
I was happy for him, of course. It is quite an accomplishment.
But it got me to thinking about how much commitment
and mental strength it requires – quite aside from
the physical strength and endurance.

I was more than impressed; I was inspired.
Oh, I have no desire whatsoever to do such a thing.
In fact, it's on my bucket list *not* to do a triathlon.
I've been successful so far in that regard;
and I'm quite confident I can make
it the rest of the way with an
unblemished record.

But, considering his feat, I can't help but wonder
just how much humans are capable of
when we put the full weight
of our desire behind it?

I highly doubt my friend thought himself
capable of such a feat ten years ago.
But obviously, he got over that.

Which proves that our beliefs about ourselves can evolve.
And so often, it's about waking up to what is possible.

It has been estimated that, for any endeavor,
what we consider our full capacity is actually
about twenty percent of our true capability.

And I'm not talking about wartime,
or in the middle of an emergency situation.
I'm talking about everyday things.

We can physically do more than we thought possible.
We can learn more than we thought possible.
We can accomplish more than
we thought possible.
Much more.

Which means, it's the "thought possible," that's the problem,
and not our capacity for doing, learning, or accomplishing things.

DaVinci said we could learn a new fact every second
for the rest of our lives, and never approach
our brain's capacity for new information.
And it's not just about information.
That's just the tip of the iceberg.

We can reach deeper levels of awareness,
develop more powerful intuition, reach levels of fitness,
and attain more financial success, than we might have
thought possible just a few years ago.
The caveat, of course, being:
We have to believe it's
possible *now*.

In terms of our limitations, our belief keeps us earthbound.
In terms of our potential, our belief allows us to fly.
And though beliefs are mostly subconscious,
it's not hard to figure out what they are.
Your life will tell you, if you
look closely enough.

If we are to reach anywhere near our human capacity for *anything*,
we will have to make the mental shift, from *"I can't,"* to *"I can."*
And while it may be a small difference alphabetically,
it will mean the difference between reaching
your full potential, or experiencing life
on a much lower level than
you were meant to.

How do you reach your full potential, or at least approach it?
It starts with deciding what you want – I mean, what you *really* want,
without all the mental chatter about whether you *can* or not;
or whether you deserve it; or the litany of other
reasons we use to convince ourselves
that something's not possible.

Humans are designed such that, if we truly want it,
it will be within our capacity to achieve it.
That's just how the system works.
The capacity for it is built
into our desire.

It *is* that simple, but most people fall short right here,
in step number one – they're not focused
enough on what they want.

Step two is – figure out what it's going to cost,
and determine if you are willing to pay the price.
Oh, it's rarely money; it's much more likely
to be time, effort, and mental discipline.

It probably cost my friend several pairs of tennis shoes,
a few sets of sportswear, perhaps a new bike,
and that's about it.

But ask him about the mental discipline it took to train
when he didn't feel like it; or to pass on the extra doughnut;
or not to quit on mile twenty when he really wanted to.
Or to ignore the constant internal pleas to stop
and do something more reasonable;
like take up fishing.

No, his feat is to be admired, simply for the strong desire,
mental discipline, and self-belief it took for him to accomplish it.
We could all do the same; but we mostly don't.

Oh, an Ironman Triathlon is not on most of our lists.
But we all *have* a list, or at least we could,
for the price of a little contemplation;
which is where the real
power starts.

What do you *really* want in life?
And what, within ethical boundaries,
are you willing to do to attain it?

Dare to Dream

Answering these will lead you to your destiny.
You just have to remember that the gap between
what you once *thought* you could do,
and what you can *actually* do,
is often a world apart.

Surely, there is no better way to say, "Thank you"
for the gift of life, than to make full use of
what you were so graciously given.'

Therefore, be daring in your dreams.
And unrelenting in your pursuit of them.
And not only will you achieve what you
previously thought impossible,
you will inspire others
to do the same.

The dreams would have been possible all along, of course.
They've just been waiting for you to dream them.

---

*All our dreams can come true, if
we have the courage to pursue them.*

—WALT DISNEY

Day 13

A Home Far Away

Because I am eternally grateful

Well, it's June 6th again – D-Day.
And my thoughts go drifting back to
my grand adventure so many years ago.

It wasn't related to World War II, not directly anyway.
In *my* lifetime, it is the day that Opa passed; a full forty-five years
after the original D-Day, which is ironic, since
in that conflict, he was a soldier
on the German side.

Many of his friends died on that day so long ago.
But Opa survived to see his family grow;
and to become part of mine
forty years later.

And every year, on this day, I look back at
what a big part he played in my life.

It wasn't likely he and I would ever meet.
But I did my radiology residency in the military,
at a time when there were still a lot of troops stationed
in what was then West Germany,
at a U.S. military hospital
not far from where
he lived.

When I finished residency, I had to go *somewhere*.
And I chose adventure; leaving a comfortable known
for the *un*known in a foreign country.
And nothing has ever been
the same.

As a young Army physician, it was risky
taking my wife and two small children with me.
It was even more risky moving to Bann, a tiny village
in the German countryside where few spoke English,
close to the U. S. military hospital where I'd be working.

It sounded like a grand adventure on the drawing board.
But once we were actually there, and I realized
there was a very real possibility of four
years of isolation, I was more
than a little nervous.

How fortunate we were to have moved in next door to Opa.
We didn't understand a word he said that first evening,
but his laugh told us everything we needed to know.
*Who tells jokes to people who don't even speak
the same language*, I wondered?

I laughed along with him, of course; but I had no idea
what he had just said. It was my first sense that we
were about to experience something special.

Looking back after all this time, and realizing how those
four years with him changed the trajectory of my whole family,
I struggle to find the words to express how much he meant to me.

He's been gone a long time now.
But it never hurts to say things to loved ones
who have passed, no matter how long it's been.
I'm convinced they hear us; and even if they don't,
it benefits us to say it to them anyway.

And for me, on this day every year, it always
seems to come down to, "Thank you."
Thank you for watching over us.
Thank you for all the stories.
Thank you for your patience as
I struggled to learn the language.

Thank you for "adopting" us into your own
family, a place we still belong, even to this day.
And thank you for making me realize
how terrible war is – for everyone.

It's hard to fathom everything that happened between that
first evening and our tearful goodbye four years later.
Even after I came home, I was never the same.
I've been home for thirty-five years now,
and he's been gone over thirty.
But it all seems like
only yesterday.

I loved him like my own father,
and I will never forget him.
Knowing him changed
Everything.

What did I learn by living in a foreign land,
and treated like family by someone who,
forty years earlier would have been
considered the enemy?

I learned that language is not a barrier to love and friendship.
"That's what the hands and feet are for," he would laughingly say,
as we half-spoke and half-played charades
to get our point across.

And sometimes, the less we understood, the funnier it got.
Language is just a tool, I realized, and often a poor one at that.
Real communication is from the heart.

It's good to experience being the odd man out, now and then;
to struggle with a new language, not know all the customs,
and have to always ask, "What does that mean?"
knowing you may not understand, even
after they explain it to you.

I learned that the word *enemy* is a convenient way
for governments to get people to do what they want them to.
And the more outrageous the stuff they want them to do,
the louder they seem to shout the word.
I wonder what would happen
if none of us listened …

I learned that people are just people.
And that flags, and languages,
and all that stuff are
just details.

I learned it's good to do something so different
that everything you thought you knew will be challenged.
We shouldn't fear it; we never lose anything of value.
It's only our false ideas that go by the wayside.
And who needed those in the first place?

I learned that traveling with your children
is one of the greatest gifts you can give them.

I learned that it says a lot about a person when
they reach out to help when you are at
your most vulnerable, even though
they have nothing to gain by it.

And when their family continues to welcome you,
even after the original someone has passed,
it says a lot about them, too.

I learned that what begins as being treated *like* family
can often progress into actually *being* family.

I learned that when you have a deep experience, it changes you.
You may think you can return to your previous life,
and that everything will be the same.
But you can't, and it won't.

Oh, you'll try, but it just isn't going to work.
It will seem like everything you knew has changed.
But, in reality, it's you who's changed.

They told me it would be hard leaving home
to spend four years in another country.
And it *was* hard, but I was
prepared for it.

What they *didn't* tell me was how
hard it would be coming back.
I wasn't prepared for *that*.

But we readjusted; and in time, made a new life,
more expanded than the old one had been.
But I've never forgotten how those
four years have changed
everything.

I don't look at flags in the same way.
I don't look at history in the same way.
I don't look at borders in the same way.
I don't look at immigrants in the same way.
I don't even look at myself in the same way;
which may have been the greatest gift of all.

It made me realize how powerful relationships are.
And how the Universe sends people to us to fill in gaps
in our lives we didn't even know we had.
That's who Opa was for me.

Looking back now, and considering how profoundly
the whole experience has changed our lives,
I literally shudder at the thought

that I might have played
it safe and not gone.

Which brings me to my final point:
Whenever you have a chance for a grand
adventure in life, it's best to take it.
Because it changes everything.

---

*The most dangerous thing you
can do in life is play it safe.*

—CASEY NEISTAT

In memory of Hermann Borst (Opa)
1914–1989

Day 14

An Off Day
Because we all have them

I had an off day today…
And I'm not really sure why.

But I gave it some thought; and for a change
I decided rather than struggle against it,
I would try to work with it as best I could.

And, I came up with the following advice,
perhaps for myself, as much as anyone else:

If you're not feeling great, don't try to do too much.
Don't put pressure on yourself to do more than you can do,
or to feel better than you feel. And above all, *don't think too much.*
Our lives ebb and flow like the tides, with a rhythm all their own.
And it's good to be in touch with those rhythms,
because there will always be things
we learn over time that don't
agree with us.

But even if we can avoid all those things, there will
be days when we think we *should* be in rhythm,
but we just aren't – and have no idea why.

There are so many factors in life,
it's impossible to account for them all.

Maybe it's the moon, or the barometric pressure,
or variations in the earth's magnetic field;
or maybe Mercury's in retrograde.
Oh, wait, it can't be that.
Isn't Mercury *always*
in retrograde?

If you're having an off day,
give yourself permission to be off;
don't give out more than you have to give;
and for God's sake, *don't focus on how bad you feel,*
since this will only make things worse.

Maybe you're not your best self today.
But you can be the best self you can be *today*.
And isn't that all that matters?

Highly aware people understand
what they have in the tank on any given day,
and don't expect any more of themselves than that.
They judge their performance that day on what they
have to give *that* day, rather than what they
have to give on their best days.

Doing otherwise will only frustrate you,
and make your off day more off
than it already is.

This is like trying to drive your car across town
when it only has enough gas to get down the street.

An Off Day

We would never think of doing such a thing, of course.
But we put such demands on our bodies all the time,
with dire consequences if repeated often enough.
We expect, even demand, that we be better than
we have the physical capacity to be.
And that doesn't make sense.

It's taken some time, but I've
started to give myself some grace
on these unexplained low-energy days.
If I can figure out it's self-inflicted somehow,
then, fine; I'll try my best not to do that again.
But beating myself up for having done it,
or wracking my brain all day trying to
figure out the cause of my malaise,
is counterproductive, and luckily,
becoming a thing of the past.

I feel off because my body needs some down time.
And without an obvious cause, it's best to leave it at that
and allow my body to have what it needs,
without complicating the process.

It's obvious our bodies need a break now and then.
They tell us this in a hundred different ways.
And sometimes, an unexplainable off day
is our body's way of telling us to stop.
So, why not give it the break it needs?
Don't plan. Don't try to figure things out.
Don't attempt to make important decisions.
If there are important things that need doing,

then by all means, go ahead and get them done.
But so much of what we *think* is important, isn't.
And much we consider urgent, can wait a day or so
until we have the energy to deal with it more effectively.

Life is about timing, I've come to understand.
There's the perfect time to do something; and there's
the timeframe in which I *think* it needs to be done.
Sometimes the two are shockingly different.

"There's a time for everything under heaven," Solomon said.
But the proper time must be felt in your heart,
not calculated in your head – *especially*
if you're having an off day.

So, if you're not feeling great, grant yourself a small vacation
and don't do anything you don't actually have to do.
Just find the best way you can to pass the time,
even if the most productive thing you
can do is take a nap.

Suit up, show up, do the things you need to do,
and do the very best you can in those things.
But other than that, let them go,
give yourself a break,
and don't make it
worse than it
already is.

Remember, you're not trying to make any headway today;
you're trying to stay afloat. So, adjust your goals accordingly.

And if you can manage to pull it off, you will find
the one thing that will make even
a down day feel better:

Peace.

And peace rejuvenates.
So do whatever it takes to find it,
most especially on an off day.
And everything else will
take care of
itself.

It's okay if all you do today is survive.

—UNKNOWN

Footnote:
A friend informed me after the fact that Mercury
was indeed in retrograde at the time of this writing,
which should be a good lesson for me to limit
my levity to things I actually know
something about.

But, then again, what fun
would that be?

Day 15

No Place Like Home

*Because you never know what you
might find right outside your front door*

I saw the trees today on my bike ride up to the clubhouse.
No, I mean I really *saw* the trees – as if for the first time.

I see them all the time, of course. But today, I really noticed them.
And they seemed more like friends than they did mere landscaping,
especially the oaks, that stretch their branches far above me
to mingle with their leafy neighbors across the street.
They're beautiful, even majestic.

It was a cascade of green, quietly escorting me to the clubhouse.
And not just green, but vibrant yellows, reds, and more;
all blending into a beautiful tapestry on this
most beautiful of mornings.

It was alive and breathing, in its own way.
And it seemed so delighted to see me;
or maybe delighted that I saw *it*.

I was here when the oaks were planted all those years ago.
They were saplings then, yet definitely more like landscaping.
But now, after all this time, they're sturdy adults.

I knew them in their infancy.
And I could say I watched them grow.

But I ask myself, *Did I really watch them?*
Did I really pay attention, or appreciate them?

It struck me that they'll be here long after I'm gone.
And though that might sound melancholy, it really wasn't.
It was more like a "circle of life" type feeling,
like all is as it should be.

There's something about living plants that feeds the human soul.
And though we tend to forget, we are designed to coexist with them.
Not only are they calming and nurturing; but also life-giving,
since they provide the very air we breathe.
And we're surrounded
by them here.

I noticed how the oaks blend seamlessly with the other flora,
some of whose names I know, most of which I don't.
But, no matter. If they could speak, I'm certain
they'd rather be appreciated
than called by name.

How many times had I passed this way over the years,
my mind in a thousand different places, worrying
about this or that – and not fully present
with the stunning beauty that lies
right outside my door?

I've always appreciated the natural beauty here – but not like this.
As I look back now, I realize it was often just a cursory nod,
from a mind largely preoccupied with something else.

Which is kind of like saying, "Yes, the Mona Lisa is a nice painting,
but I really have to get to the grocery store before it closes."

But today, I saw more deeply. And I realized that it was
always here for me – if I had taken the time to notice.

It dawned on me that the drive from the gatehouse to my home
might be the most beautiful stretch of road in all of Naples.
And I admonished myself for driving it back and forth
for thirty years before ever having that thought.

But admonishment is never appropriate I reminded myself.
We can only function at our level of awareness at the present time.
No one should require more of themselves than that.

I'm just glad that my awareness got a little deeper this morning,
on this ride to the clubhouse I've made hundreds of times.
And I'm grateful for it, because my life just got richer
without having to actually go anywhere.

We truly live in a visual oasis.
And when you in add the symphony of the birds,
and the small furry creatures scurrying about,
the wonder of it only deepens.

This oasis has greeted me every morning for years.
But what I realized *this* morning was:
My life is a lot richer when
I greet it back.

There are lots of beautiful and interesting places in the world. But for those of us fortunate enough to live here, there truly is no place like home.

Everywhere we look, the complex magic of nature blazes before our eyes.

—VINCENT VAN GOGH

Day 16

What Will They Say?
Because it will change the way you live

My mom passed recently; and needless to say,
I've been thinking about it a lot lately.

I miss her, of course, but she was in her nineties,
suffering from dementia, and basically ready to go.
It's always sad, of course, for those left behind,
even when the passing is an expected one.
But there was nothing to be done.
It was just her time.

After the funeral and the family gathering were over,
and all the Mom stories had been laughingly told,
I found myself contemplating my *own* mortality.

Oh, I'm not concerned about taking my turn when the time comes.
But I can't help wondering: What will they say about *me*
when it's all said and done, and nothing
can be added to my story?

They'll likely not speak of my possessions,
since those will be possessed by someone else;
death making a mockery of the idea
that we can ever really
possess anything.

And my achievements, also made in the world of form,
will quickly fade once I pass to the other side.

My job was important, as I judged it, a real service to others;
a place where I made a difference. But they'll get along
fine without me, just like they did before me.

And the children? They were so much more important;
my only real legacy, when all is said and done.
It might be said I did a good job with them,
but there will be holes they'll have to
dig themselves out of because
of my shortcomings.

No matter how hard one tries, parenting is
one of those jobs that just can't be done perfectly.

So, hopefully, they will take that into account.
And when they look back, they'll do so in kindness,
consider the abiding love I had for them enough;
and find some sort of peace with the rest.

But, regardless,
as soon as the funeral is over,
they'll go back out into the world,
where they'll be judged by their own actions,
and not by who their father was.

The real question, though, isn't what they will say.
But rather, what would I *want* them to say?
This needs to be my main concern,

since I'm still here, and have
some time yet to affect
that conversation.

So, what would I like to hear concerning the life
I will have just concluded if I were sitting
unnoticed in the back row,
a fly on the wall,
so to speak?

I was proud of the job, and of the achievements.
And I was particularly proud of the children.
So, a few words about these would be nice.
Maybe more than a few about the kids.

But all things considered,
when the hourglass is finally empty,
and there's nothing more I can add to the story,
if they say I was a lover of God,
I will be content.

And that I was willing to grow, and develop
a larger view of what that actually means
than what it meant when I thought
I had it all figured out.

And that I was willing to face my inner demons,
and do battle with the darkness, even when it was hard.
Even when there were battles lost.

And that I did the necessary self-examination
to be able to love better at the end
than I did at the beginning.
And to find compassion
when it was not easy
to come by.

And that I never quit trying.

Beyond that, it's all details, it seems to me.
Does it trivialize things to distill a well-lived life
down to just a few short paragraphs,
when life is so complex
and mysterious?

No, I think not.
The simpler, the better.
Because it's actually *living*
those few paragraphs
that matters.

It's a worthwhile exercise to figure out what
you want people to say about you at your funeral,
then go about living your life so as to make it happen.

Yes, this is a good thing;
set up the target, far in the distance;
then live your life so in the end, you hit it.
It will change the way you live,
which will change what they

say about you when
you die.

Oh, it will no longer matter to *you* what they say.
But it will matter to them. And to leave them
with beautiful words to say when
they think of you
is a gift.

It's not a *material* gift. But it will be your *last* gift.
And, in the long run, perhaps the most meaningful.

The purpose of life is not to be happy.
It is to be useful, to be honorable,
to be compassionate, to have it
make some difference that you
have lived, and lived well.

—RALPH WALDO EMERSON

Day 17

Precious Moments
Because they're all we really have

I watch the moments go by, fleetingly,
one after another, after another.
And then they are gone.

They pass in front of my eyes before
I can even reach out to grab
hold of them.

Gone before I can even grasp their significance;
some seemingly important moments, not a big deal at all.
And other seemingly mundane moments that grow
in importance the second they fade into the past.

A walk with the grandkids to buy ice cream.
A silly game, made up on the spur of the moment.
Uncontrolled childish laughter, over I can't remember what;
only that it was shared with me. Yes, this is the important thing.

It was shared with me.

What will the grandkids remember
when they think of me years down the road?
Will it be the sweet memories I'm making with them now?
Or some other random events I can only guess at?

I remember my own grandfather, whom I adored in so many ways.
Was he aware he was planting memories that would remain
in my heart long after he had passed from the scene?
At the time, I just loved being with him.
He was caring, funny, and safe,
and seemed to genuinely
enjoy my presence.

If there are other requirements for being
a wonderful grandfather, I don't know of them.

And, yes, I think he did know, even at the time.
The passing years have a way of giving us perspective
that is impossible for us to have as a child.

When we're a child, our only job is, well, to be a child.
It's the adult's job to think of all the other stuff.
And, if we're in touch with how life actually works,
part of that job is to realize how fleeting it all really is,
and enjoy it the best we can while we're actually living it.

Yes, this is of prime importance.
Because it all goes by so very, very fast.
Time spent with family, especially the little ones,
allows me indirect influence on a future I will never see.
And, long term, what could be more meaningful than that?

To the untrained eye, it may look like a silly game, or a walk to
the store, or playfully helping with Italian homework
when I don't even speak Italian; but

none of that is the point.
It's what I plant in their heart that matters,
as my own grandfather taught me so very long ago,
without ever having uttered the words.

Being around children is a joy. Their innocence is disarming,
and the requirements to be accepted are so minimal.
You just have to meet them on their level,
be willing to give of your time,
and genuinely care.

That's the easy part.

The hard part is watching the present become the past
so quickly it makes your head spin, without
the power to do anything about it.

Oh, I'm sure on a cosmic level it all makes sense.
If I had the power to pause these precious moments
and hold on to them, I'm sure they'd be diminished somehow,
though it doesn't stop me from wishing I could.

But, since I can't, I'll just have to accept it's this way for a reason,
and make the most of each moment as it presents itself,
knowing how fleeting they all actually are.

The only antidote, it seems,
is to enjoy them as they're happening,
appreciate the memories, which I get to keep,
and continue making more.

Which means, that there will be more laughter tomorrow,
and more silly games, and who knows what else?
It's the not knowing that adds to the
adventure of it all.

What will they remember of it,
years down the road? Who knows?
That's not for me to say.

I only know that spending meaningful time with them now,
gives me a chance to be part of their treasure chest of memories
that they will accumulate over their lifetime.
And if that's not time well spent,
I don't know what is.

Moments, as it turns out, are all we have.
And, at the end of the day, all we have to give.
So, make each one count, is my advice,
in any circumstance, certainly.

But if you have any to spend on
the little ones in your life, don't hold back.
Because, in the long run, those moments will be
the most beautiful and long-lasting of all.

---

*Life is a series of memories
that once were just simple moments.*

—UNKNOWN

Day 18

Anonymous

Because it doesn't matter if anyone knows

I did a small thing today
and helped somebody out,
even though I didn't have to.
And it made me feel really good.

Oh, I try to be helpful whenever I can.
So, it's not like it's never happened before.
But I'm surprised how much this time affected me.
I canceled a medical test someone didn't need, that's all.
I didn't expect a Nobel prize or anything. It *is* my job.

And it wasn't even an invasive test.
There would have been no side effects;
just extra time and expense for the patient,
not to mention the hassle and the needless worry.
It's the type of thing I always feel good about doing.

I make lots of important decisions in a day, some of them life-altering.
But this wasn't one of them. So, why was it such a big deal today?

I went out of my way to do it, for one thing.
I wasn't in the decision loop, in terms of the initial test.
I was asked after the fact if I could
take a look and help out;
and so, I did.

And, I found myself in the right place, at the right time,
with the right credentials, and the right experience to make the call.
Which in this case, was to call the whole thing off.
Because it just wasn't necessary.
And she'd already been
through enough.

How sure was I?
One hundred percent,
or I wouldn't have made the call.
But, again, why did this time seem so different?
Maybe it was the seeming anonymity of it all that struck me.
I'm not her primary doctor, I'll likely never meet her,
and she'll probably never know who I am.
I don't do my job for the "Thank-you's,"
but there was never going
to be one for this.

And there were more important decisions I made today, for sure;
although, if asked, this person would probably beg to differ.
But I'm still trying to come to grips with why this
particular good deed struck me so much,
when my job is all about
doing them.

Maybe it's the combination of things:
That it wasn't life-altering in a major way,
and seemed sort of random in my day,
and that the one who benefited,
will never know it was me.

Yes, all that, plus how darn *good* it made me feel,
has made the whole thing seem pretty remarkable to me.
It's certainly a reminder that good deeds are their own reward.

It's been said that we are judged by how we treat
people who cannot benefit us in any way.
And, perhaps even more so, being
of benefit to those who will
never know about it.

And even though the one affected by today's decision
likely *will* never know, and will never know *me*,
we will always be connected in some way.
That's just how things work.

The recipient of my decision will be
forever affected by it in some small way.
And I will be forever affected by having made it,
even though the two of us will never meet.

But isn't it *all* like that?

If we're all interconnected, can there even
be such a thing as an isolated event?

How many people had a role in producing
the book you're holding in your hand?
It was a lot more than just me.

And where did the paper come from?
How many trees? Who cut them down?

How did they get to work? Who paid them?
And what about their families?

No, there is no such thing as an isolated event.
The ripple effect of everything we say and do is real.
And just because we can't trace the ripples
doesn't mean they're not important.

Everything we do affects the human family in some small way.
And the more we keep this in mind, the more we will
consider our actions before we take them,
and our words before we speak them.

Which is wise, because the ripples our actions create
don't get *too* far down the road, before
they wash over us as well.

Therefore, be kind,
whether anyone finds out about it or not.
Because, at the end of the day, you are the recipient
of your own kindness, just as much as the one you gave it to.

You know, it seemed like such a small thing I did today.
But, the more I think about it – maybe it wasn't.

Remember, there is no such thing as a small act of kindness. Every small kindness creates a ripple to which there is no logical end.

—SCOTT ADAMS

Day 19

Mistakes

Because they're going to happen

"It doesn't have to be perfect," the teacher said.
"If you're not quite sure how to do things,
take your best guess, start doing it,
and you'll figure it out from there.
If you wait for 'perfect,'
you'll never get
started."

I was taking an online class about finding one's purpose.
Oh, I've had a meaningful career; and certainly,
being a physician is part of why I'm here.
But I've always felt I had more
to offer the world
than that.

Akyiia, the class leader, is quite intuitive.
And when she says something,
there's a sense of it coming
from a deeper place.

Which is probably why her words made so much sense to me.
And might explain why I've been having so much
trouble getting started on this next
phase of my life.

And then it dawned on me:
Maybe the thing I've been avoiding
is exactly what I should be doing,
which is – making mistakes.

Yeah, that's it. Maybe I've been looking at it wrong
by trying to avoid something that not only can't be avoided,
but also may be a hidden secret of success – *just start making mistakes*.
They're going to happen anyway, so why not embrace them?
The only way to never make a mistake
is to not do anything, which is
the biggest mistake of all.

If your goal is to avoid mistakes, you might as well
say goodbye to your dreams, because you're
not going to realize them – ever.

Perfection is not just the enemy of
your dreams – *it is the enemy of your soul.*

Fear of making mistakes leaves you at the starting gate,
watching others who don't mind making them
run a race that you were always
meant to run, too.

Every general knows no battle plan survives the first shot.
And the victor is not the one with the best initial plan,
but the one who is the most adaptable once
the chaos starts – and life is no different.

Don't wait until you have a perfect plan.
Make a good plan. And begin with that.

Then, go ahead and make your mistakes.
They are not to be avoided, but embraced.
Because it's impossible to learn without them.
Make them; make them willingly; and rejoice in them.
Because each one will bring you closer to your goal.

Thomas Edison didn't find the correct filament
for the light bulb until his one-hundredth try.
He wasn't any smarter than his colleagues.
He worked harder and was more persistent.
He was unmoved by the ninety-nine "failures,"
considering them instead, stepping stones to success.
He never took his eyes off the "light" at the end of
the tunnel, rather than staring at the
tunnel itself, which is always
only darkness.

So, celebrate your mistakes, because they mean that you're trying.
Consider them road signs, guiding you to your destination.
Trust me, once you've arrived, the number of
turns it took you to get there will be
completely immaterial.

The one who makes the most mistakes always
learns the most. And the one who learns the most,
in any endeavor, is usually the one who wins the prize.

The real key is not in *avoiding* mistakes;
it's in not making the same
ones twice.

The following is a foolproof formula
for success in any endeavor:

Start making mistakes, and start making them now.
Try to always be making different ones.

Always look forward, and not backward.
Focus on the light, and not the tunnel.
Never let the goal out of your sight.

If the word "failure" comes into your head, don't listen.
It's okay to be discouraged from time to time. Just don't quit.

And, most importantly, enjoy the process.
If you can't make it fun, then stop;
find something that *is* fun,
and do that instead.

Life is too short to do otherwise.

Mistakes are part of the dues one pays for a full life.

—SOPHIA LOREN

Day 20

Hi, Mom!

Because they're never really gone

I thought about you today.
And I miss you …

Oh, I don't want you back.
It was too hard on you at the end.
And I know you wouldn't want to make
a return trip either just to go through *that* again.

But I miss you all the same.
Mostly, just that you were always there,
in your quietly supportive way, that never had to
announce how supportive
you were.

And how you always thanked me for calling or stopping by.
And how happy it seemed to make you when I did.
It's hard to put a value on knowing that
someone's always glad
to see you.

It's pretty simple, though not everyone has that figured out.
But you did. It's relationship genius, really.
The simple things often are.

And you were always such a great listener, too.
Which was another simple thing you did.
You listened, and you always cared,
but never told me what to do;
even when I wanted
you to.

You always allowed me to figure it out on my own,
which is just something great parents do.
And, I guess I miss that too.

What?

I can still talk to you anytime I want?
And you'll listen to me just like you used to?
And you're still a fan, even from where you are now?

I guess I do still feel your support, now that I think about it.
And most of the support I felt from you here was
when I wasn't physically with you.

Yes, I know you still won't tell me what to do.
I knew that was a useless pursuit by the
time I went off to grade school.

But I'll take you up on your offer from time to time, if that's okay.
I guess it makes sense I can still feel you if I pay attention,
since the time and space thing no longer affects you.

And, thanks for everything you did,
though I know I told you that
while you were here.

I appreciate more and more how you wanting me to be
honest, hard-working, and kind, but not caring about the details
beyond that continues to help me navigate this life.
I doubt I'll get it all figured out down here,
even by the time I come to join you.
But you gave me a
heck of a start.

I always felt lucky on the mom front, even when I was little.
Yes, whenever they were handing out moms,
I definitely got in the right line.

You did so many of the simple things so well.
And the complicated things, the window dressing kind of stuff?
Well, I've learned all that on my own, and you were right:
It's fine in its own way, but wasn't really
important in the first place.

Anyway, thanks again, for everything.
I miss you – but it's nice to know
I haven't really lost you.

What we have once enjoyed we can never lose;
all that we deeply love becomes a part of us.

—HELEN KELLER

Day 21

An Opportunity

Because a positive outlook is always best

A temporary job came up recently that I would like to do:
a Center for Mind-Body Medicine training in Ukraine.
The work is needed, and I'm on the faculty,
so, it's possible I can go – perhaps.

It's beautiful work, heartfelt work;
helping traumatized populations learn
to heal from all the trauma and the stress.
And then teaching them how to teach others,
so that the process is self-sustaining.

It is truly life-changing for everyone involved.
There could be no better use of my time and effort.
But not many faculty will get to go.
Only a few will be chosen.

I've not been active with the Center recently,
and haven't done as many trainings as other faculty.
And though I'd like to think I'm good at it,
I don't do group work for a living
as many faculty do.

No, there are others with
far greater expertise than I.

And yet, I *am* on the international faculty.
And *have* gone to other places with them.

And I *am* a physician with military experience,
which could come in handy in a war zone.

And I'm generally pretty calm in uncomfortable,
chaotic, and even dangerous situations;
which could also come in handy
in a war zone.

So, there you have it,
reasons they'd choose me to go,
and just-as-valid reasons they wouldn't.

But, the bottom line is, Ukraine's heart is bleeding.
And though I can't fix it, I can help in some small way.
It seems I'm needed there, and I deeply want to go.

So, I decided to handle this situation
differently than I have such things in the past;
and see if I could consciously create the opportunity,
rather than wringing my hands over the issue,
feeling confident about it on my good days,
and down on my doubtful ones.

So, I've focused only on positive thoughts about it.
I see myself there in my mind's eye, and more importantly,
I feel myself already there deep in my heart.

And I not only see it happening,
but see it as *already* having happened.

And it feels wonderful.

I've taken the lists of the *Why They Would Want Me,*
and *Why They Wouldn't,* and narrowed it down
to consider only the *Why They Would.*
And that, in itself, feels great.

I've applied for many things over the years,
some of which I've gotten, and some not.
But the waiting process has always
been a mixed bag – sometimes
calm and confident,
and sometimes
not.

So, I decided that *this time,* I was going all-in,
and started planning the trip, telling others I was going,
and just all around started *feeling* myself there.
Previously, I would have considered
how foolish I would look
if I were wrong.

But, *this* time,
I just … didn't … care.

And do you know what?
The experience has been wonderful.
A much-needed break from past patterns.

I now know what they mean by,
*"seeing what you want in your mind's eye,
and rehearsing it so intently, that you
feel ahead of time like it's
already happened."*

And if we can manage to pull that off,
our hearts are open, and we're truly grateful
*for something that hasn't
even happened yet.*

Ah, but has it?

Which raises the deeper question of whether
our internal reality is more real
than the external.

There is a lot of evidence that this is exactly the case;
and that the external world is just a physical
manifestation of what's going on
in our hearts and minds.

And, if this is truly the case,
most of us have a lot of work to do
in rethinking how things actually work.
Because it's much different than we thought.
And we are more powerful than we
had any idea we could be.

But getting back to the matter at hand,
after a few weeks of purely positive intention,

and refusing to consider the negative side of things,
I had convinced myself that they did, indeed, need me.
And that the reasons I shouldn't go weren't nearly
as important as the reasons that I should.

I had convinced *myself*, was the final result.
And I felt great about it, and confident in my abilities,
which is so very different than my past
experiences with these things.

They haven't chosen yet. That will be in a few weeks.
But I truly feel that I have won this game.
I was my biggest fan and advocate.
And it's hard to put a
price on that.

If I don't actually go, that will be perfectly fine.
It's been a wonderful experience already, though I am
convinced I'll be taking the trip soon.

But the biggest question
as I contemplate all of this, is:
If it was so wonderful not listening to
the long list of my shortcomings,
and refusing to entertain the
thoughts when they
did come up,

Why can't I do that all the time?
Wouldn't that be a joyful existence,

whether I got exactly what
I wanted or not?

Because at the end of the day,
manifestations are just manifestations.
And material is just material.
It's the joy that's
the thing.

Which is exactly what we get when we
insist on viewing ourselves in a positive light,
despite our occasional missteps and mistakes;
and leave the negative thoughts alone to
churn and stew amongst themselves,
in the sewer from whence
they came.

Leave them alone, I say. Let them be.
They seem to be happy there.
No need to elevate them
by giving them space
in my head.

What would life look like if we refused to listen to:
I'm not good enough, and *I don't deserve it?*

Take some time to consider, because it might be
hard to imagine anything quite so grand.

These are just thoughts, at the end of the day.
With no power to harm us until we grab
hold of them and believe in them.
The choice is wholly ours.

So, am I going to Ukraine? I hope so. I think so.
But it doesn't matter; because either way,
I've clearly already won this game.

---

*Intentions are like magnets; the more we declare them,
believe in them, and act in ways to manifest them,
the more powerful and real they become.*

—UNKNOWN

Day 22

Frustrated

Because we've all been there

Wow, the mammography techs were frustrated today.
And I felt for them, though their frustrations were system-related;
so there wasn't much I could do about it, other than lend an ear,
listen as empathetically as I could, and try to help
them see the bigger picture.

I did my best to talk them off the ledge, as it were,
having been there many times myself, and
remembering how grateful I was
to have someone listen.

It wasn't a major issue, just an ongoing thing
where they get caught in the middle from time to time.
Work-related systems don't function smoothly all the time.
There are glitches in even the most well-run companies
that can complicate even the best of jobs.
And, every once in a while,
we just need to vent.

So, I was happy to catch the exhaust today,
and chat with them a while until things calmed down.
You might say it was a kind thing to do, and I suppose it was.
But pragmatically, I'd also hate to lose a couple of valued techs to
actually *jumping* off the ledge over a temporary frustration

that they'll be better able to handle tomorrow
after a good night's sleep.

It was a nice conversation, and though,
again, nothing was solved, at
least they know I cared.

But, it got me wondering about frustration.
What is it, actually? And how do we best deal with it?
We've all been there, after all. It's part of the human equation.
So some deeper thought on the subject might be helpful,
since it isn't going away any time soon.

It seems to me we get frustrated
when we see things not working right.
It's a good thing, as I've always understood it.
I mean, we all want things to work correctly, right?
We desire a smoothly-running system which follows
the rules or guidelines, whether that's a work situation,
or a relationship, or having the trains and buses run on time.

But, now that I think about it, I'm wondering what universe
we're talking about, because when has that *ever* been the case?
Things *always* go wrong, and people are *always* doing
what they shouldn't, or not doing what they should.
Which means, that apparently on some level,
we think that simply by being frustrated,
something's going to change.

Good luck with that.

Our frustrations serve as a warning to us: that something
needs changing (if we are in a position to change it),
or if it *can't* be changed, that we need to
make peace with it – or remove
ourselves from the
situation.

We *could* stay in an unchangeable situation, and allow ourselves
to be chronically frustrated. But this is not skillful living
as the Buddhists say, since it changes nothing,
and degrades our health in the process.
No, this is not a wise choice.

Frustration, at the heart of it, is a call to action.
It is a signal from our soul that something is amiss.
The problem comes when we use the signal device as a *tool*,
thinking that somehow our frustration alone will change things.
But frustration over things we cannot change is like
beating our heads against a wall, hoping that
the wall is somehow going to move.
And we all know how that goes.

Yes, we're using our heads, but there are better uses for them,
like choosing to temporarily put our frustrations aside
and taking time to connect with our hearts,
which then allows us to use our
heads more wisely.

This is our place of power, and our place of clarity.
But we will never find it as long as we let
our frustrations go unquestioned.

Our frustrations *always* have a message for us; but ironically,
we cannot hear the message in the midst of the frustration.
Once we are at peace, we will not only know what to do,
but will also make use of the proper tools to do it.
The powerful know they can effect change
by prayer and positive intention alone,
with much less effort, and
no heartache at all.

Hoping to effect meaningful change by frustration alone
is like using a cart and a donkey; while making use
of prayer and positive intention is like using
quantum physics to do the same job.

The latter, though unseen, are *infinitely*
more useful than the former,
and a lot less messy.

So, when frustration calls to you, give it its due.
There will be life information that will be helpful to you.
But once you hear the message, let your frustrations go quickly.
And see them as the light shining in the darkness that they really are,
lighting a path for you to go elsewhere, or lighting one inward,
helping you to better understand yourself
and grow into who you were
always meant to be.

And whether you leave or stay, or take action or not;
remain at peace always, and return to it quickly when you lose it.
This is your center. This is your power. This is your wisdom.

Rejoice in it. And live *from* it. And you will
always know the right thing to do.

In this world so full of imperfection,
we cannot ask for more
than this.

Your mind is like this water, my friend; when it is agitated it becomes difficult to see. But when you allow it to settle, the answer becomes clear.

—MASTER OOGWAY

Day 23

Am I Smiling?
Because we could all do more of it

"Yoga should be fun," my teacher told us.
"In fact, if you can't smile while you're in the pose,
then you probably shouldn't
be in the pose."

We all chuckled a bit, but it did make me wonder:
Do I smile while I'm in my yoga poses?
I had to admit, I didn't know.

And since yoga is a metaphor for life,
it follows that I have no idea in
the rest of my life either.

How much do I smile?

It's certainly worth some deeper thought.
I mean, my yoga teacher smiles all the time;
and I know some others who do, too.
And they all seem pretty happy.
Coincidence, possibly?

Probably not, I thought to myself, smiling.
Then I thought back to all the "smilers" I have known.
They had to be doing it on purpose, right?

I mean, nobody's *naturally* that
happy, are they?

But if the smilers are all happy, why isn't *everybody* doing it?
A good question, I decided. Why do people *not* smile?
Maybe smiling is a signal that life is good;
and for many of us, we think
life has to be harder
than that.

Certainly, we live in a *no pain, no gain* culture,
where nothing is considered of value unless
it was accomplished by hard work.

If you don't believe me, all you have to do
is go to the gym, look around, and see
how many people are smiling
while they're working out.

I can save you the time,
because it'll be pretty close to zero.
And why do they call it *working* out, anyway?

Sure, it's only the gym, you might say, but it's deeper than that.
Because how we do *anything*, is how we do *everything*,
which in Western culture, means we try to muscle
everything and make it bend to our will,
even at the price of possibly
injuring ourselves,
or others.

But life is meant to be easier than that.
Because if we're trying to muscle everything,
we completely leave out the unseen dimension,
which was always meant to be part of the equation,
and is always working on our behalf;
if we wait long enough to
give it a chance.

Understanding that we're not alone in anything we do
means we can relax; knowing if we do our part,
there is another part that's being done *for* us.
This not only takes the pressure off,
but makes everything fun.

This is exactly why people with a
spiritual perspective on life smile so much;
they know they don't have to do it all by themselves,
and thus, they enjoy the ride so much more.

It's not *no pain, no gain,* anyway. It's *no discomfort, no gain,*
discomfort being oh, so very different from pain.
It's through discomfort that we grow:
physically, mentally, emotionally,
and spiritually.

Pain warns us we're being injured, nothing more.
It's the fire alarm in the building, crying,
Stop what you're doing, right now,
because something needs
your attention.

Discomfort, on the other hand, is a promise;
of an expanded future, with even greater possibilities,
if we just *keep on* doing what we're doing.

Pain and discomfort sound similar, but they're a world apart;
the point being that we can *smile* through discomfort,
and learn to *breathe* through it, while contemplating
the future growth that will surely come out of it.

So, I think I'll try smiling a lot more.
And not just in yoga, but everywhere in life.
Smiling is self-medication, at the end of the day,
because we feel good immediately after we engage in it.
We self-medicate with so many other things,
why not do it with something that's
actually good for us?

So, I decided that, going forward, no matter what I'm doing,
I will check in with myself, and see if I'm smiling.
And if *not*, then ask myself, *Why?*

And along with that, a daily self-awareness exercise:
How often do I smile, and can I raise the
percentage just by paying
attention?

All of which is deeper than we think; because our smiles
are not so much about how the world sees *us*,
but about how we see the world.

And for the price of a simple smile, we can make it more beautiful today than it was yesterday. Which is the *real* power of a smile.

Because of your smile, you make life more beautiful.

—THICH NHAT HANH

Footnote: Just to satisfy my curiosity,
I took a straw poll among friends and family
to see who smiles when they're frustrated.
And these are the unofficial results:
(names omitted for my personal safety)

Yes: 0%
No: 10%
Hell, no: 10%
I have no idea: 80%

Yep, that's pretty much
what I thought.

Day 24

A Troubling Memory

Because childhood memories aren't that reliable

I made an appointment to see a publisher today.
And my memories drifted back to so many years ago …

I've always loved writing, even when I was little.
It was the first thing I ever loved doing;
before sports, or girls, or travel,
or any of those things.

When I was nine, I put a collection of my stories in a
Kleenex box and tried to send them off to be published.
I didn't want anybody to find out for some reason.
But somehow Dad did, though I'm not sure how.
Maybe it was the taped-up Kleenex box that
I stuffed in the mailbox with no postage,
and the words *To the Publisher*
on it that gave it away.
Who knows?

I just remember my dad coming down the stairs,
box in hand, and how my heart sank when I saw him.
This is not going to go well, I remember thinking.
But there was nowhere to escape, so
I just stood there, waiting …

"Nobody's going to publish those,"
I remember hearing him say.
I was crushed, of course.

I felt embarrassed, humiliated, ashamed.
*I **knew** that's what he'd say,* I remember thinking.
That's why I didn't want to tell anyone in the first place.
I won't ever put myself out there like that again.
Not until I can do it all on my own.

And how could he brazenly crush
a little kid's dreams like that?
It just felt so mean.

But life moved on, and sports happened, and girls;
and with the passage of time, I quit thinking about it.

What were the stories about, you ask?
Oh, just short stories. I only remember one:
The Battle of the Hot and Cold Planets,
including some colored drawings
of the battles I had imagined.

But I'm pretty sure all the other ones were the same:
about *some* kind of war, intergalactic or otherwise.
I have to admit, even now, it's pretty intriguing.
I mean, who could ever win such a war?

Do ice rays freeze heat rays, or do heat rays melt ice rays?
The answer will be forever lost to history, I guess.

I have no idea what became of
the Kleenex box.

Suddenly, my musings were
interrupted by a voice in my head:

*"Hey Tommy, how about I go with
you to your appointment?"*

It was Dad!

Why would he even say that after what he did?
But the voice sounded genuine, and as my heart softened,
I did remember him saying something like, "Just wait a few years."

Yes, it didn't all seem so harsh now, as I revisited the memory.
It probably crushed *him*, now that I think of it, to have
to tell his creative, hopeful, and innocent little boy
that it just wasn't going to happen.
And he was right, of course.

I felt love in my heart for my dad,
as I now saw the memory though adult eyes,
rather than those of a wounded child.

*Sure, Dad, come along with me.
I'd love to have you there.*

It all felt so wonderful, now – so clean.
Kind of like I had my dad back.

And it made me wonder – how many *other*
childhood memories hadn't happened
exactly like I remember them?

I mean, Dad came off a lot better after a second look.
Who else might benefit from a comprehensive
review of the stories of my wounded past?
Probably lots of people, I imagine.
But the *real* benefit would
have to be for me,
would it not?

No matter who we are, our lives unfold along the storyline that
we tell ourselves about who we are and why we are here;
which is largely based on memories of early life events,
regardless of whether or not the stories are true.

Thus, we only have to change the story
in order to see our lives change dramatically.
I can't change what happened to me in the past.
But I *can* change the way I remember it now.
And isn't that basically the same thing?

But back to the present: What about my
upcoming appointment with the publisher?
Well, I think it will go beautifully.

How can it not, with Dad, my biggest fan, right there beside me?
But, Dad, you said "a few years," and it's been nearly a lifetime,
I said, lamenting the long passage of time since

A Troubling Memory

I first wanted to change the world
by what I write.

"Ah, Tommy, those things are unknowable," he said.
*"But whenever it does happen, it will be the perfect time.
That's just the way it works."*

I see, I said, trustingly.
*Well, we're here together, now;
so, whatever it turns out to be, will be
good enough for me.*

It felt good to have my dad back.
It was a warm, comfortable, safe feeling.
Who knew such a thing was even possible,
given that he passed away decades ago?

Such is the magic of questioning your memories, I suppose.
It's never too late to rethink things, or to remember differently.
Beautiful things can be uncovered, or *recovered*,
for the price of a little contemplation,
and keeping an open mind.

Take the journey.
It's *well* worth the price.

---

*All memories fashioned at the level
of a child's eye, are unreliable in scale.*

—CAROL O'CONNELL

Day 25

Disappointed
Because it didn't happen like I thought it would

Well, they chose the faculty to go to Ukraine.
And I *was* on the list, but only the wait list,
and buried at the bottom of it at that.
It's not a *complete* impossibility.
But it's pretty darn
close to that.

So, what do you do when you're disappointed?
When you were pretty sure something
was going to happen, but didn't?

Well, the main thing is to realize that sometimes the story
is more complex than you thought; and sometimes
the story's not over when you *think* it's over.

So, be sure to wait until it's *really* over before
declaring it over and moving on. That's number one.
And number two is: If it's *truly* over, and you didn't receive
what you expected, trust that things happen for a reason,
and that Spirit has your best interest at heart.
Because it always does.

How many times have you seen people lose jobs,
only to find a better one shortly thereafter?
Or found a great relationship, after

losing the one they had, not
by their own choosing?

So, even when the story's over,
it's still not over, because there's always
a much bigger picture that has to play out.
If things are truly done, and the passage of time has
clearly made it impossible for your vision to come true,
look at it as a *chapter*, and not the whole story.
There is always more to play out.
And the overall picture is
larger than you can
comprehend.

It's about trusting that things are working out for you,
even though at the moment, you may not be able to see how.
It makes short-term disappointment easier to deal with – keeping
mild disappointment from becoming *bitter* disappointment.
It's not a problem to recover from the former.
It's easy to get stuck in the latter.

Mild disappointment says,
Okay, maybe my ideas were a little off,
but let's see how it all plays out.

Bitter disappointment says,
Because it didn't happen the way I wanted,
all is lost, or worse still, *Nobody cares about me,*
or possibly even worse, *I didn't deserve it anyway.*

Disappointment will happen from time to time.

It's part and parcel of the human equation.
But regardless of our disappointment,
there *will* be a new tomorrow.

And the mildly disappointed will have a huge leg up
over the bitterly disappointed in meeting that tomorrow.
Because one meets tomorrow from reasonably level ground,
while the other has to climb out of a self-imposed hole.
There is nothing wrong with being disappointed.
It means you're living life, and that you care.
Just don't hang out with it for too long
because it will cloud your view
of the bigger picture.

The bigger picture is always there, so work hard to find it.
It will make sense of your disappointment in time.
And often turns disappointment over an event
into *gratitude* for the same event, once you
finally see how all the pieces fit.

And when that happens, it's a beautiful day;
because the *next* time you have an expectation
that doesn't quite pan out, you can smile,
and enjoy the even bigger surprise
just around the corner that
you can't quite see yet.

That's when faith and trust become fun.
And disappointment can be seen for what it is:
a small bump in the road, on the way to

something better than what you
originally had in mind.

Did I feel a bit foolish being so completely all-in
on something I really wanted, but just didn't pan out?
A little, at first. But holding to a positive outlook
the whole time was such a good experience,
it far outweighed the small bump
in the road when it
didn't happen.

No, I can't say I'm sorry about any of it.
All-in is better than playing it emotionally safe,
even if it did turn out I was wrong.

They say, when you think positively, positive things happen.
And now that I think of it, isn't that exactly what happened here?
I thought my experiment was a failure, because it
looks like I won't be going to Ukraine.
But, from a larger perspective,
wasn't it a rousing
success?

Something very good *has* come out of this;
which is a template for how to handle future desires:
Be unrepentantly all-in, no matter what anybody thinks.
And be relentlessly positive concerning your desire.
Don't allow any negativity to enter your head.
Just see what you want, and *only*
what you want, in your
mind's eye.

And then be at peace with whatever happens, because from that place, disappointment will be no more than an occasional cloud passing overhead.

And then *every* day is a beautiful day.

---

*Don't let today's disappointments
cast a shadow on tomorrow's dreams.*

—UNKNOWN

Day 26

A Long Overdue Goodbye
Because time is not the barrier we once thought

I had a dream last night
about my childhood dog, Lady.

She was old, and lying in bed,
barely aware of her surroundings.
A few weeks went by with no change,
and we all knew it was just a matter of time.
It seems I had a say in whether to let her
go peacefully, or to let her
linger for another
week or two.

And, though I didn't want her to go away,
I agreed with everyone that she was suffering,
and there was no point in prolonging the inevitable.

Suddenly, I realized it was a dream; but the dream didn't end
like it usually does when that happens. It's called lucid dreaming.
You're aware it's a dream, but you can continue the dream anyway.
It's the same dream, except you can guide it now if you wish.
It doesn't happen often, but I love it when it does,
because profound things always happen.

And I decided, since I now had a say, that *this time*
I was going to tell my beloved dog goodbye,

unlike the first time, when I had
no say at all in the
matter.

I looked into her soft brown eyes,
and said, *Goodbye, Lady. I... love... you.*
You've been the best dog a boy could ever ask for.
And I will never forget you, even if I live to a hundred.

I didn't see her pass in my dream, but it didn't matter.
I'd had my time with her that I didn't get
to have so many years ago.
And I felt complete.

Then I thought back to Mom and Dad. Yes, they should have
told me, but honestly, what were they going to do?
They knew wrestling was important to me;
and they didn't want to upset me.

I do still think it was the wrong call.
But it was made out of concern for me.
And how can I complain about that?
Looking back, it makes me realize
just how much I was loved.

It was emotional, saying goodbye to Lady,
but not as emotional as I would have thought.
She had grown old and frail, and who
knows how aware she
was of anything?

It was just her time, and that's the way of things.
There was nothing to be done – only to say goodbye,
and appreciate the time I had been
given with her.

It was a sweet dream and time of contemplation afterward.
And as I looked back at my memories of a time long past,
I realized that what they say about the past isn't true:
You *can* go back. You *can* change the memories
of your past, and feel more whole today.

Oh, you can't actually change what happened.
But you *can* change how you react to the memories,
as well as imagine better endings. And
isn't that the same thing?

It's a type of healing.
And a type of forgiveness.
And we'd be wise to make use of it,
since we can do so consciously,
with a little mental effort.

Did I get to say goodbye to my beloved dog?
Well, maybe not back in the day, but I have now.
And who's to say which "reality" is more real?
I'm at peace now when I think about
her passing – and isn't that
all that matters?

Some say time doesn't exist, except in our heads.
While others say past, present, and future
are all happening at the same time.

Which, if true, means that the so-called past
may be more malleable than we thought.
And forgiveness, a more creative act
than we might have imagined.

The past may be set in stone from one perspective.
But if we have the power to remember it
from any perspective we choose,
why not choose one that's
more palatable?

Why not choose the healing salve of a larger perspective,
rather than holding on to our wounds like they
were a badge of courage of some kind?

They say that we create our own future, and so we do.
But we can *re-create* our past in the same manner,
using a different lens to look back with,
and refusing to focus on the
negative aspects.

It's not just what happened to us, after all.
It's the story we tell ourselves about it that matters.
When we're small, we think there *is* no story; there's just us.
But later in life, with growing awareness, we realize
it's just a story – and stories can be changed.

My story is: I loved my childhood dog deeply.
And I got to see her off while learning
a bit about life and death
in the process.

And my parents loved *me* deeply,
and missed the dog every
bit as much as I did.

So, what's the problem?
There isn't one.

Not anymore.

---

*We are products of our past, but we
don't have to be prisoners of it.*

—RICK WARREN

Day 27

The Magic Flute

Because late is always better than never

The music in my home as a child was practically zero.
It wasn't forbidden; it was just never encouraged.
So, I decided early in adult life, that someday
I wanted to play a musical instrument.

And I had always loved the flute,
so I knew the flute was going to be it,
whenever the "it" came to pass.

And then, life happened:
medical school, the military, kids,
living overseas, returning home, more kids,
moving out of state to take a civilian job;
and then a life of basically work
and kids' ball games.

So, before I knew it, decades had passed,
and I hadn't given it a second thought.

But *one day*, upon realizing that the kids were now gone,
and that "someday" can actually be code for "never;"
in one of those *if not now, when?* moments,
I decided it was finally time.

So, I started online flute lessons.
And this is how it went:

It was humbling, first of all, to be a grandfather,
and not able to read a single note of music, or have any
idea of rhythm, or what a key signature is, or know
what all the dots and lines actually mean.

I have advanced degrees, and am quite experienced
in my line of work; yet here I was, learning the alphabet
all over again, and sometimes finding myself
quite frustrated by my lack of progress.

It didn't help when Amanda, my online teacher,
helping me learn note values, said,
"Think of it this way,"

"Quarter note – eighth note – sixteenth note:
Bread – je-lly – pea-nut-but-ter.
That's what I teach my
second-graders."

"Thanks, Amanda," I said, "that's very helpful,"
while my already-fragile ego cringed
in the corner, begging
her to stop.

Suddenly, I had a mental an image of myself
sitting at a child's school desk, feeling conspicuous
and uncomfortably out of place among a classroom of
second-graders, whose desks seemed to fit them just fine.

Interestingly, the second-graders didn't even notice,
apparently considering me just one of them.
That's kids for you, I thought to myself.
*They're way more accepting
than we are.*

As time passed, my ego got used to its newly-diminished role;
I resisted the rough patches when I was tempted to quit;
and these are some of the things I've learned:

A flute is just a hollow metal tube with holes.
It's a *vehicle* for the music, but it's
not the actual music.
I'm the music.

Which means:

That posture matters. A positive attitude matters.
Breathing properly matters; and eating the right things;
and drinking enough water; and keeping my stress level down.
Though I've never told her, Amanda is like a mix
between my mom and my yoga teacher.
And, she's right, of course.
Just like they were.

It's almost as if I, *myself,* am just a vessel for the music.
And the more relaxed I am, and the better I
take care of myself, the better
the music will be.

I almost said the better music I will *make*.
But if I'm a vessel, that means I don't
really "make" the music, right?

And, if the flute's just a vehicle, and so am I,
then *where does the music come from?*
And why do we love
it so much?

It's worth some contemplation, given that the vibrations
of the music are the same as those of the flowers,
and the birds, and the trees.
And the stars.

Some maintain that the first words that
created the universe *were a song*.
It doesn't get deeper
than that.

Yes, it makes the music seem more mystical, and magical,
and more beautiful than I had considered it before.
And I found myself both wistful about how much
I had missed by not discovering it earlier in life,
and grateful that I had discovered it now.

No, it's not "just"' music; it's a miracle – and a gift,
like so many other things we take for granted.
And the lessons such things have to teach us
in our pursuit of them are gifts as well:

Like, making mistakes is part of the process.
And that if we're not making them,
we're not learning anything.

That visualizing success leads to success,
while focusing on our shortcomings
just makes it all a struggle.

That there will be good days and bad days.
And it's best to enjoy the good ones,
and tolerate the bad ones,
knowing another good
one can't be too
far away.

That trying too hard is counterproductive.
And that striving for perfection is a waste of time.
That you can't force a musical instrument to do *anything*.
And you can't wrestle it to the ground and conquer it,
because it will just end up conquering you.
That the way to ultimate success
is time-tested and true:
Keep showing up.
Keep trying.
Don't quit.

And the best lesson of all:
That music is supposed to be fun.
And if it's not, you aren't doing it right.

I've been at it for a couple years now, and I'm a lot better.
I might be up to fourth or even fifth-grade level now.
I could check with Amanda at my next lesson;
but, honestly, I'm afraid to ask.

If you ever decide you want to learn a new skill later in life,
I highly recommend it, as there are a myriad of benefits,
even beyond what I have mentioned above.

But if you do, take my advice:
Check your ego at the door, because
if you bring it to class with you,
it isn't going to be happy.

Live as if you were to die tomorrow.
Learn as if you were to live forever.

—MAHATMA GANDHI

Day 28

The Inner Critic
Because we all have one

Well, the day's almost here.
It's off to the publisher's tomorrow.
And we'll see where all this goes.

How do I feel?
A little annoyed, honestly,
that it's taken so long to get here.
What's held me back? Me. Only me.
There's no one else to blame.

People have complimented my writing for a long time now.
But somehow, I never seem to quite believe them.
Or I believe them for five minutes, and
then go back to my default
internal assessment:
It's okay.

Why just okay? Because it's attached to me, apparently.
If somebody else had written the same stuff,
I'd probably be raving about it.

I find myself wondering if it's possible
to assassinate one's Inner Critic.

It sounds harsh, I know,
but that's where I am with it.
Oh, I suppose it's never good to
want to kill any of our inner voices.
But I'm sick and tired of this one.
So could I at least tie him up,
gag him, and sit him
in the corner?

Where does he come from, anyway?
Why does he wield such power over me?
He criticizes everything I think, say, feel, or do,
simply because I'm the one thinking,
saying, feeling or doing it.

Oh, we all need an Inner Arbiter;
you know, some inner sense
to let us know whether
we're on track
or not.

But it needs to be judged fairly,
and not so obviously skewed toward
the negative that it's
ridiculous.

It's like having my own personal "East German judge;"
you know, the one who at all the Cold War-era Olympics
gave out the most absurdly negative scores.
Except for the East German
athletes, of course:

English judge: 8
Spanish judge: 9
Swedish judge: 10
Venezuelan judge: 9
Saudi Arabian judge: 9

East German judge: 3

It was downright laughable at the time.
But it's less so now, when I realize that guy
is alive and well in my head and never lets up.

I wonder again, *Who is he? Where does he come from?*
And, more importantly, *How do I get him to shut up?*

I suppose he's an echo of sorts, from back when shame was
the preferred method of child-rearing, coaching,
making sure you got to class on time,
and a thousand other things.

Oh, it works as a motivational tool, I suppose.
Fear of the consequences makes you want to
avoid the consequences. I'll give you that.

But there's a heavy price to pay when
we carry that voice with us into adult life,
and have a hard time getting it out of our heads,
mistaking its critical voice as our own,
and the lies it tells as the truth.

Anything we do is considered less-than,
just because we're the ones doing it.
It's never going to be good enough,
because *we're* not good enough,
is the unspoken message.

Who am I to write a book?
Who am I to change the world?
Who am I to... *(fill in the blank)?*
You'll *never* be the one,
as long as you listen
to the voice.

And, trust me, it doesn't matter *how* accomplished you are,
or how many times outcomes have proven the voice
to be wrong. It's still there telling you that
you can't, or that you shouldn't.
Or that you're not
good enough.

You can't kill it, as much as we'd all like to.
It does seem to have free access to the human mind.
So, as a matter of practicality, we're just going
to have to find a better way
to deal with it.

But how?

The simplest way to look at it is to ask ourselves,
What is the nature of the voice? And then,
What tools do we have to deal with it?

I think we can all agree, first of all, that the
voice of the Inner Critic is not one
that has our best interest
at heart.

If we consider the baseline healthy human state as loving
and open-hearted, with all our energy systems running
smoothly and synchronously, then we could
look at the voice of the Inner Critic
as "foreign" to us, in a sense.

It is not a healing voice; it is not a soothing voice.
It is a diminishing voice, a demeaning voice,
sometimes even a destructive one,
and *always* a false one.

It doesn't add any value to our human hardware.
Quite the contrary, it only gums up the works,
which is completely predictable because
when we listen to its voice,
we just feel bad.

In this sense, the voice of the Inner Critic is like
a "ghost in the machine," or a software virus
that infects our delicate human hardware.
It's there, running in the background;
but it's been there so long that
we no longer even notice.

And this is where our power begins – once we notice.
And once we *do* notice, our next level of defenses kick in:

the power of our belief, and our power to choose.
If we use these wisely and confidently,
we can crush the Inner Critic
beneath our feet.

And we can do so every single time.

The Inner Critic has the right to speak.
But we have the right to not accept the message,
believe otherwise, and to choose a different direction.
And once we do, its hold on us begins to fade,
no longer being fed by our agreement
with its demeaning stories.

It's profound, but it's not hard. And it all begins with an awareness
that the message is garbage to our souls, and is best resisted.
Nobody buys apples at the grocery store without picking
through them and putting the rotten ones back.
Shouldn't we question the voices in
our head at least as closely?

Following these simple steps is life-giving:
Be aware. Don't believe every thought
that runs through your head.
Keep the healthy ones,
and throw the
rest back.

The key is remembering that *you're* in charge
of your Inner Critic, and not the other way around.

I even talk to mine sometimes.
And when it hands me the same-old:
*"Who are **you** to change the world?"*
I have a standard reply...

*Who am I **not** to?*

Winning the war of words within your soul means learning to defy your inner critic.

—STEVEN FURTICK

Note:
If you get really good at this,
you better buckle your seatbelt, because
without this voice to hold you back, there's no telling
where you might be off to, or what you could accomplish.
It's what naturally happens when we put ourselves
back in our mental driver's seat, where
we were always meant to be.

Day 29

Graduation Day
Because we can all find our way back home

Today was one of those magical days
when it seems like you're floating on air.
Except I've not had any days like this before.
Oh, I've had magical days – just none quite like this.

I had my appointment with my publisher today.
And even before I left the house, I had the feeling that,
no matter how it went, my life would never be the same.

It reminded me of the day I received the
letter from the only medical school I had applied to.
I stared at the letter for some time, not opening it for a while,
realizing that the contents of it would change my life.

I wasn't nervous; I would have been fine being turned down.
There were plenty of other interesting things to do in life,
and I was sure I'd be able to find one of them.
But it was a yes, and the rest is
history, I suppose.

And today seemed kind of like that.

Thinking back all those years ago to the Kleenex box,
and fast forwarding to now, it seemed

my whole life was finally
coming into focus.

But why had it taken me so long?
Why did I doubt myself so much along the way?
Was it just a ridiculously circuitous path,
or was it always meant
to be this way?

None of that matters now, I decided, as I backed the car
out of the garage; not even worth considering at this point.
Just like on med school acceptance day, I wasn't at all nervous.
They'd either love what I write or they wouldn't.
And that would be that, I figured.

The fifteen-minute drive there was surreal.
Odd as it might sound, I'd swear the trees were
cheering for me as I drove to the gatehouse – *wildly.*
The entire way, they cheered as if it were graduation day,
or I were walking to the stage to be given some kind of award.

And it moved me to tears. I found myself being grateful that
I had finally discovered them those few weeks ago.
They were friends now; I greet them every day.
And now they were giving back.
And it was beautiful.

Once outside the gate, the rest of the trip was no less magical.
I wondered if I should have sent them a different set
of writings to review, perhaps better than
what I had initially sent.

It doesn't matter, said an inner voice.

I even took a wrong turn, to a location
I know very well, and feared I might be late.

It won't matter, said the same voice.

And I continued driving in perfect peace.
It almost felt like I was headed to my destiny,
and no detail, great or small, was going to change it.

Well, I arrived on time, and met April, the publisher,
and Heather, the head editor, and both were delightful.
And, of course, they loved what I had sent them,
which you have probably guessed
if you're now reading this.

"You must have felt like you were ten feet tall,"
a friend said to me as I was telling the story.
"Not at all," I replied. "It just seemed normal."
As I believe it would have felt if they *hadn't* liked it.
Being unattached to outcomes is a beautiful place to be.

The two-hour meeting was over before I knew it,
and I was on my way home, trying to wrap my head
around everything. It all seemed so much larger
than whether I ended up with a book or not.

It was hard not to think back to that shy little boy,
who was so convinced he had something worthwhile,

he tried to sneak it to a publisher without telling anyone.
And then, suddenly – I saw everything differently.

I thought back to the moment my dad
began walking down the stairs, box in hand.
Wait a minute, I thought, that little boy felt ashamed
*before his dad ever got to the bottom of the stairs,
and before he had ever uttered a word!*
That incident wasn't the problem.
It was indicative of a
deeper problem.

There had to be a family culture
that had caused him to be so secretive,
so untrusting, so unwilling to be vulnerable.

And, then it all came flooding back…

True, it was "Leave it to Beaver" on the surface.
And yes, there was lots of family fun and laughter.
But laughter can also be used as a weapon
when it turns to sarcasm and ridicule.
And laughter should *never* be used
as camouflage for such things.
Especially as it concerns children.

I realized that my childhood home had been
physically safe; but wasn't always emotionally so.

Of course, that little boy was going to
write stories all about wars and battles.

On the surface it was mostly fun and games,
but underneath, it could be an emotional war zone.

Some children push back when they don't feel emotionally safe.
But sensitive children often hide – sometimes for a lifetime.
They live life in plain sight, even quite successfully.
But the real them lies hidden away,
somewhere deep within,
where it feels safe.

Oh, this isn't a knock on Mom or Dad.
Most family traumas are generational in nature.
No one is unscathed; so, it's up to us to understand the
larger picture, appreciate how much Mom and Dad
protected us from, and heal from the rest,
so we ourselves don't pass it on.

Suddenly, I saw movement just
ahead, in the shadows.

It was Tommy.

Oh, my God, I thought.
He sees me… and knows who I am.

I called to him, as gently as I could, fearing he might run away;
and he inched his way a bit further out of the shadows.
We looked at each other for a few moments,
as if for the very first time.

It was a tender moment – one that I'll never forget.
Then I took a chance, and broke the silence.
"Listen," I said, "I understand where
you've been, and now, I think
I finally understand why."

"I'm going to ask you to come with me, if you're willing.
Yes, I'm more experienced in the outside world,
but I need you as much as you need me.
We're better together."

"It's not much of a life for you there in the shadows,
cut off from the rest of the world. I know you feel safe there,
but that time is past, and you have too much to offer the world
to stay there forever. It needs you. And I need you; so please come."

"Remember when you didn't try out for the school play,
even though you desperately wanted to, because
you were afraid they'd laugh at you?"

He nodded, tentatively. Yes, he remembered.
It was clear that the memory still bothered him.
"Well, we have a voice now; both of us, together.
And it will be bigger than the school play.
And I promise you, no one will laugh."

"Think about it," I said, reasoning with him.
"People won't spend money on a book they don't like;
or even waste their time talking about it. They'll just put it
down quickly and move on. And we can live with that, right?"

He nodded his head again, and made a funny face.
He was warming up, I could feel it.
He knew I had a point.

"Tommy, your Kleenex box made it to the publisher today.
And they *loved* it. So, let's do the rest of this together."
His face brightened ever further now,
and he ran up and gave me a hug;
maybe as deep a hug as he'd
ever given anyone.

"Well, there will be lots of hugs from now on,"
I said to him, reading his thoughts. "I promise."

"But why did it take so long?" he asked trustingly.
"Ah, Tommy, those things are unknowable," I said,
repeating my dad's words. "I only know that whenever it
happens, it's the perfect time. That's just the way it works."
Yes, it seemed that things had come full circle.
And now, perhaps finally… I was home.

---

*There is a part of every living being that wants
to become itself; the tadpole into the frog,
the chrysalis into the butterfly, the damaged
human being into a whole one.
That is spirituality.*

—ELLEN BASS

Day 30

The Rest of the Time

Because we all need a power source

People think I have it all together
because I write this stuff.

But I don't.
Well, I *do*, actually,
but only while I'm writing.
The rest of the time I have to
slog it out in life just like
everybody else.

You'd think I have the secret of happiness at my
fingertips, and never worry about anything.
But, sadly, that's not how it works.

If I seem to have it together while I'm writing,
it's only because I'm plugged in while I'm writing,
nothing more – but nothing less, either,
since this is not in any way
to be diminished.

In fact, as near as I can tell, our experience of life
is largely determined by whether we
are plugged in or not.

And we can't just plug in once.
We have to continually plug in to
have any real power in life.

Plugged into what?

To Source, however we understand it.
To the Unseen Realm that connects all things,
knows all things, and will speak to us,
if we're willing to engage
in a conversation.

We are created such that we need to continually
take in something to survive on this planet.
And whether we thrive or not, depends
on what we choose to take in.

On the most basic of levels, we have to have air.
We must breathe every minute of every day, for a lifetime;
or, by definition, that lifetime will come to an end.
After we breathe, some of the air molecules
quite literally become part of us;
and it's the same for
food and water.

Thus, we *are* what we take in.
And what we consistently take in
determines how well
we will live.

We ourselves determine the "what" and "how much."
The choice is always ours, and ours alone.
And the physical quality of our lives
will be borne out in
our choices.

As will the spiritual quality of our lives,
which underlies and affects
everything else.

Which brings me back to the writing.
Because for me, it's just a way to plug in,
hear a voice wiser than my own – and to listen.

And the more consistently I return to the well,
the better off I will be, since I can no more make one
peak experience with the Divine last a lifetime
than I can sustain life from one meal,
a single glass of water, or
one breath of air.

Trust me, when your consistency drops off,
your patience, generosity, and the
quality of your relationships
all start to head south.

If I don't breathe, I will soon suffocate.
If I don't eat or drink, I will starve or die of thirst.
And if I don't feed myself spiritually, though my spirit won't die,
it will go into hibernation, which is basically the same thing,

with all the attendant consequences (see above).
That's just the way it works.

So, yes, I write these. And I'm in the center lane when I do;
feeling in touch with a wisdom greater than mine,
which I can then use to enhance my life,
and hopefully, in the reading of them,
enhance yours as well.

But I have to constantly re-read them.
And continually engage in new conversations.
And take to heart what I hear; and do my best to apply
it to whatever shows up in my life every day.

This leads to a powerful life.
At least that's been my experience.
It's *my* life; but it's not my power, ultimately.
Rather, it's something I am privileged
as a human to tap into,
if I choose.

Sure, I'd like to take credit for the writing.
And yes, it *is* my hand and my pen, so to speak.
But I could no more come up with all this on my own
than a toaster could produce a piece of toast
without being plugged into the
outlet on the wall.

The power outlet is available to everyone.
That's just how the human system is designed.
And the best thing is, when you're plugged in,

you can relax, and trust what's within you
to take care of things in a way that
you could never figure out
with logic alone.

There is tremendous peace in that.
And you don't have to understand it any more
than you understand the power that
comes out of the wall.

You just have to learn how to work with it.
And if you don't know, all you have to do is ask.
It will not be withheld from you.

To say it's worth the effort is a gross understatement.
Because Source will infuse its power into whatever you do.
And once you experience that, you will see how
the deeper dimension influences *everything*.

And life will never be the same.

---

*A connection to Spirit restores your confidence,
relieves your anxiety, and relieves you from the desire
to control everything in your life.*

—SONIA CHOQUETTE

Day 31

A Labor of Love

Because it's always good to say yes

I was riding my bike this evening, just to get
in some movement and enjoy nature, as I often do.
And it dawned on me that this project is almost done.
Just a few finishing touches, and then that will be it,
as far as my part of it. And I had mixed feelings.
I'm a bit melancholy that it will soon be over.
But am deeply grateful to have participated.
My request had been granted, it seems;
that I would be a *vessel* for this book,
and not the actual Author of it.
There's great peace in that.

To say it's been a labor of love
would be the grossest of understatements.
To spend so many hours in deep contemplation,
able to ask any question I wanted, without being judged,
is to be in the safest of places, in the most
Loving Presence you can imagine.

Sometimes I got answers, sometimes not. But it never mattered.
The questions are the main thing I've learned, not the answers.
Open-ended questions are the playground of the Divine,
with the only variable being: Do we want
to play along or not?

We miss a lot if we don't.
Because the discoveries are as
profound as they are unpredictable.
For me, it was like hunting for Easter eggs,
finding them and bringing them home, only
to discover that they were deeper parts
of myself I never knew were missing.

I wasn't searching for anything in particular when I started.
But what I found was more precious, *and* more personal,
than I could have imagined in the beginning.

As I rode further, I looked up into the always-beautiful evening sky,
and through tears of gratitude, said, "Thank you. For all of it."
"But why did you choose *me* for this project?" I asked,
feeling deeply humbled by it all.
"Why choose *me*?"

"I chose many, Tom," came the brief reply.
"You're the one who said yes."

When I say yes to life, life says yes to me.

—LOUISE HAY

Conclusion
Always a Surprise

I didn't intend for this book to be *my story,* but that's the way it turned out. As things progressed, and I realized that this *was* my story, I briefly considered changing it, but thought better of it. *Of course, it was my story,* I realized. And it was *always going to be* my story. I just didn't realize it until all the pieces came together at the end.

Once you make a commitment to look deeper at the everyday things all around you, you'll start finding messages in them, and the messages will be specific to you – the exact ones you need at the exact time you need them. You won't see a pattern at first, but there always is one, and as you continue to follow the breadcrumbs, you'll start to see it. And if you *keep* following them, it will lead you to exactly where you need to be, knowing exactly what you need to know, when you need to know it.

You might see similarities to my story, or you might not. And though the details will differ, the principles are the same, since the human journey is common to us all. If you're willing to follow, you will be led on a journey all your own. The destination? Unknown. The hallmarks of the destination? Powerful. Beautiful. Profound.

Every path, if followed deeply enough, leads to the Divine. And a hallmark of the Divine, however we understand it, is wholeness. Thus, the closer we get to it, the more whole we become. We won't have to ask; it just happens.

This is why spiritual seekers don't care if they seek forever; because there are always deeper levels of understanding, which lead to deeper levels of wholeness – which allows us to see deeper still. It's the upward spiral of all upward spirals. And once you find the path, you never want to stray from it.

So, do you want to find the secrets of life? Just start looking at the simple things around you – and look inside you. Examine your memories. Question them. Comfort them, when need be. And the profound will never be far behind. Because what we so often don't take into account while searching for it is; it wants to be found, even more than we want to find *it*.

Yes, hide-and-seek seems to be God's favorite game; but in this version, the One who's hiding actually *wants* to be found. Which may explain why it always hides in plain sight – because it makes it that much more fun.

God has created the world to play hide-and-seek with man.

—KEDAR JOSHI

Putting it All Together

The following is a brief synopsis of the main points of each daily reflection. When you've read each reflection enough times that it's second nature to you, you may find it helpful to go through this "Cliff Notes" version as a reminder of the main focus from each day. Seeing all of the main points written down together will help you integrate them into your life. Review them often – we all need reminding.

1. Forgiving your parents is the only way to ensure that you don't end up doing the same things they did. And if you already have, forgive yourself, and you will receive a double benefit. Whatever it was, just let it go. They were doing the best they could.

2. Our primary relationships are the greatest source of our stress – *or* healing. Work hard to make sure they are healing. It will help you live happier and more productively everywhere else.

3. Forgiveness is mandatory if we are to reach our full human potential. We're all like hot-air balloons, and every unprocessed wound is a rope keeping us earthbound. Release them, one by one, no matter how long it takes – and set yourself free.

4. Curiosity, wonder, gratitude, love – all reasons enough to live in the present moment. Oh, there are a multitude of other reasons, but these four remain. And the greatest of these is love.

5. The beauty of nature is a healing balm for our soul. Contemplate it often. It will help you understand your place in the great Mystery.

6. The human mind has the capacity to make even the most magical of things seem boring if we let it go unchecked. Don't let it go unchecked.

7. What we believe – about ourselves, and the world – is the biggest determining factor in the kind of life we lead. Make sure your beliefs are working *for* you, and not *against* you. When we stop believing in our own limitations, they tend to disappear. And when we believe we can fly – we do.

8. Pay closer attention to the other sentient beings who inhabit the planet with us. They are no less miracles than we are. Honor them. Appreciate them. Protect them. They have much to teach us, if we're willing to learn.

9. Gratitude is a superpower. And it's no more than a habit. Work to cultivate the habit. It will enhance your life more than you can imagine.

10. Trial and tribulation exists in every life, but so does humor. Find it as often as you can. It makes everything easier.

11. Think about your long-term friendships from time to time, even if they're not active at the moment. Celebrate them. They were a gift, no matter how long they lasted. They're always just a memory away, and can bring a smile to your face whenever you decide you want one.

12. We are happier and more productive when we have a dream for the future. If you don't have one already, find one – and make it big. If it scares you a little, you're probably on the right track.

13. How does it work that people come into our lives and heal us? It's a mystery. I only know that whenever I think of them, it makes me smile, I am grateful, and I feel loved.

14. If it weren't for the *down* days, we would never recognize the *up* ones. Thus, down days are a necessary part of human existence.

Learn to honor them. You can fly again tomorrow.

15. In your rush to meet the future and your search for new adventure, don't forget what's right in front of you. It's more than you think – and much deeper.

16. Remembering that we won't be here forever is one of the greatest catalysts for a happy and productive life. Remind yourself of it daily. It is an antidote to wasting time, taking things for granted, and losing perspective.

17. Understanding the connection between today's moments and tomorrow's memories is a profound awareness – one that puts you squarely in charge of your future. Build it wisely.

18. Every kindness you do, no matter how small, benefits the human family in some way. So, be kind, as much as you possibly can – without regard for personal benefit. We all need it.

19. The truth about life is, we're all just muddling through. So, make peace with it, and you'll be a lot happier. If making mistakes were the end of the world, the world would have ended a long time ago.

20. Our loved ones who have passed are never really gone; our physical senses just can't perceive them. But our deeper senses can. Love doesn't die when we do; so remember them. They remember you.

21. A consistently positive outlook on life is another superpower. And, like gratitude, it, too, is just a habit. Work to cultivate the habit. You will be glad you did.

22. Listen to your frustrations, and do what they ask of you – change something, change yourself, or leave. Then, let them go. Do this, and you will meet them as a friend with a valuable message. Otherwise, they'll just seem like a hassle.

23. The more you smile, the better you feel, and the better the world looks to you. Do it a lot. You owe it to yourself.

24. Not everything in our life happened exactly like we think it did. Question your memories. Strive to see them from a different perspective. They *affect* your life, but they shouldn't *rule* your life.

25. Expect the best, but hold your expectations loosely. Sometimes the best turns out to be better than you imagined – and later than you thought.

26. According to Einstein, the distinction between past, present, and future, is a persistent illusion. And if so, healing our past by choosing more pleasant images to carry around in our heads about it, may be easier than we think.

27. Never stop learning. It keeps you young, and makes you more interesting.

28. Take mental control over your Inner Critic, and you will take control of your life. This, also, is no more than a habit. Work to cultivate the habit. Things will be a lot quieter in your head – and more peaceful in your life.

29. The formula for a happy life is simple: Find the thing you love to do; and do it as much as you possibly can. That's it. Everything else will take care of itself.

30. The overwhelming majority of reality is beyond the ability of our physical senses to perceive. This is not in any way metaphysical; it's a cold, hard, scientific fact. So, learn how to cooperate with the unseen. It only makes sense; and it changes everything.

31. The Universe sends us many invitations, in many different ways. And we say "no" more than we realize. Practice listening. It's a matter of *wanting* to hear, more than anything else – then make it a policy to say "yes."

Going Deeper

*The discipline of writing something down
is the first step toward making it happen.*

—LEE IACOCCA

The following are 31 daily exercises to deepen the experience of each day's reflection. While the reading and rereading of the reflections themselves is the main goal, taking the time to go through these exercises will deepen the process. Many of the exercises call for making lists; go ahead and make them, even if it takes you a while. Don't feel obligated to finish each list the same day. The exercises will likely blend into each other as time goes on; and since everything is interconnected anyway, it doesn't make any difference. If you find yourself on Day 23 for instance, and something comes to you to add to your Day 12 list, by all means, go ahead. It's not meant to be a rigid process, because life doesn't happen that way. If you think I wrote these in order, you would be wrong.

    Look at the exercises as an ongoing practice. You will never be truly finished with them, because life is always evolving. So, enjoy the process, and don't be too concerned with keeping things to the actual day. Eventually, your ever-evolving lists will become a greater resource than the initial writings. If you stick with the process, the changes over time can be profound.

Day 1 The Ladder of Life

Gratitude or Grace ...

Our childhood memories continue to shape our lives well into adulthood. It's fun to celebrate the wonderful ones, but also important to find grace for the harder ones, realizing that we're all just doing the best we can. Make two columns; label one Gratitude, and the second one Grace. Then go down memory lane and consider experiences from your childhood family of origin. Assign each memory to a column. Either it was something you are now grateful for, or it was something difficult that you now need to find grace for. Only two columns – that's all you get. It's okay to use shorthand for each memory. Just a phrase or two that brings an event to mind is fine.

Don't go to particularly traumatic memories at first. Start with small things and build from there. The Gratitude list, in particular, will help in dealing with the things on the Grace list. Don't feel like you have to forgive something that you're not ready to forgive. It's just an exercise to help you see where you are with everything. And to gain perspective.

Which list fills up more quickly; Gratitude, or Grace? If the Grace list fills up first, which is common, just work a little harder on the Gratitude list. How different do you feel when the Gratitude list starts to catch up? Pay attention to how you feel. It's like mining for gold in terms of understanding yourself and your relationship to your past.

Day 2 Returning Home

We can always do better ...

Consider your current family dynamics, whatever they might look like. Even if you don't have any blood relatives, you still have a metaphorical family – be it friends, colleagues, or teammates. Just identify who they are, appreciate them as such, and consider the dynamics. What's going well? What would you like to change?

Whatever the state of your current family, things can always be improved. So, that's your task today. Even if things are good, how could they be better? Focus on yourself, not them: What could *you* do better? And then resolve to do it. But be careful; the status quo is always a lot more comfortable. Find the courage to break the mold, and do something new. After doing the Day 1 exercise, you might see your own family dynamics through a new lens.

Day 3 A Long and Winding Road

A list to heal your soul ...

Make a list of the people or experiences that you have not yet forgiven. Sit quietly and simply ask yourself; "What haven't I forgiven?" Keep asking, and make a list. Writing it down brings our thoughts into the manifested realm, and this will help.

Don't worry about actually forgiving at first. Just write down and acknowledge the places you are still holding on. Once you've acknowledged it, the forgiveness will come in time. The list won't let you forget. That's the magic of it.

Day 4 The Last Drop

Now is all we have ...

Today, pay full attention to the present moment and the smallest of things; brushing your teeth; watering the plants; driving your car; a conversation. Do your best to lower the volume of the background noise in your head. Focus intensely on what you're doing and nothing else, as if the world didn't otherwise exist.

In a conversation, try to hear every word the other says without internal commentary. Focus on them, and *only* them, and see how that works for you. Then give the same attention to everything else.

Day 5 A Peaceful Evening

Be curious ...

Today, be curious about everything. Ask questions; especially open-ended ones, to no one in particular. See what answers come, and how they come. You will eventually get to a place where the answers end – which is where wonder begins. Keep asking questions until you get there. It's a beautiful place. Nature is great to start with, because it doesn't take many questions before you begin to feel the "bigness" of it all. But it doesn't have to be nature. Many are the roads that lead to wonder. Take any one of them you like.

Day 6 A Mundane Day

Everything is important …

Today, consider everything important, no matter what it is. Don't think about outcomes; just the thing in front of you. Pay attention to how you feel doing each thing. Do it with the utmost care. This has the power to change your perspective and make each day endlessly fascinating. Even if a task is not really important, *pretend* that it is. That will make it fun.

Day 7 The Placebo Effect

An overlooked source of power ...

Take some time today to focus on the overlooked, but obvious, message of the placebo effect – that people recover from even serious illness, *just because they believe they will.* You're welcome to research it if you like, it's well-documented. The numbers vary depending on the condition, but roughly 30 percent of *all* conditions are either improved or resolve entirely due to the placebo effect; *which means due to a person's thought and belief alone.*

Take some time to consider: If your focused thought and belief are powerful enough to bring about physical healing – without any medicine at all – what *else* might they do? That's your question for the day. It just might be the question of a lifetime.

Day 8 A Boy and His Dog

A love letter …

Think of your most beloved pet, either current or a previous one. Then write a brief letter to it telling it how much it means/meant to you. The more time you spend on it, the deeper the experience will be. If you've never had a pet, ask a close friend to describe their relationship with their favorite pet – present or past. Make it a good friend, who's willing to go deep with it. And then be willing to listen to them closely. Ask questions. You could learn a lot; about the animal-human bond, as well as your friend.

Day 9 Grateful

The bus is waiting ...

Imagine that this exercise is the last thing in life you will ever do. Don't worry; it won't be. But for educational purposes; let's pretend it is. You get to finish this writing exercise, and that's it. The bus to heaven is right there waiting – no getting out of your chair; no phone calls; no Get-Out-of-Jail-Free card. You get to finish the exercise; and that's it.

Once you've set the mental tone, write a few notes to people in your life you have been grateful for – and tell them why. The notes don't have to be long; they just have to be heartfelt. Even just a few lines is fine. Then make a list of other things you have been grateful for: experiences, events, abilities, or even just life itself.

Coming to terms with our mortality has a way of driving us to gratitude. So, take the ride – and enjoy it. Let it sink in for the rest of the day (it turns out you *did* have a Get-Out-of-Jail-Free card). Maybe find a way to share your notes with those most important to you. It will mean the world to them.

Day 10 The Pizza Guy
Take a break …

Today's a freebie. We all need one from time to time. Just relax, think about how the whole process is going, and be grateful for any positive changes you're experiencing. But otherwise, just chill for today. Maybe order a pizza...

Day 11 An Old Friend

Reach out ...

If you were to call an old friend you haven't seen for a while, who would it be? Why not call them? Don't call on their birthday or a holiday. Make it a "just because I was thinking about you" call, without any agenda. You might rekindle an old friendship and you might not; that's not the point. Just call as a celebration of what was; nothing more. And see how it makes you feel.

Day 12 Dare to Dream
What if…

What would you do if you knew that your capacity, for anything, was 80 percent higher than you previously thought? What would you attempt that you otherwise wouldn't? Give it some serious thought, and start a list. Then go about making the top things on the list happen. You can jump-start the process of manifestation by assigning a tentative time frame. Your self-confidence will get a huge boost when you accomplish them. And you will inspire others as well, so it's a win all the way around.

Day 13 A Home Far Away
They changed everything ...

In every life, there are a handful of people who changed everything. Not counting family, who are those people for you, and what have they meant to you? There may be some overlap with your gratitude list, but these are people who have had a profound impact on your life. Yes, you're grateful for them – but it's deeper than that.

Spend some time today contemplating how much of a difference they made in your life. And if they're still with us, find a way to tell them. They probably know they have helped you, but they may not know the depth of it. Find a way to let them know; it will mean the world to them. If they are no longer on this plane, write them a letter. Take the time to express yourself fully. It will be a beautiful experience, I promise.

Day 14 An Off Day
Be prepared ...

Think of things you do that add to your overall well-being, and that just make you feel good. This might include biking, walks in nature, meditation, listening to music, and so on. But don't forget basic self-care things as well; things that are so simple we normally don't even think of them: brushing your teeth, drinking enough water, taking your supplements, taking a nap, or time in the pool. *The smallest things matter,* because on your off days, you won't have the energy for most of the normal things.

Make two columns – label one Normal Days, and the other Off Days, and then start writing things down. It's important to make separate lists, because it takes into account the normal variation in how we feel on any given day. Sure, you feel fine today, but you *will* have off days, and on those days self-care is going to be hard to come by. On those days, every small thing you do for yourself will lift your mood ever-so-slightly – and sometimes that's all you need.

Make sure to have your Day 9 gratitude list nearby. It will come in handy. The key is to be prepared when an off day comes, because they come at unpredictable times. Think of it as reviewing your emergency procedures at home or work. You don't wait for the emergency; you do it ahead of time. And that's what today is for.

Day 15 No Place Like Home

Find magic right where you are …

Take the time today to notice things in or around your home you usually don't notice. There is magic everywhere. Once you start looking, it won't be hard to find. It could be something grand, or it could be something incredibly small, like a memento, or even a houseplant. See it in a new way. The deeper you look, the more you'll appreciate it. If you do this every day, you will soon find yourself deeply appreciating things you barely noticed before.

Day 16 What Will They Say?
There's still time …

Write your eulogy. That's it. Not what they *might* say now. But what you would *want* them to say when the time comes. Include multiple perspectives; your partner, children, friends, co-workers, and so on. Once we're gone, people *want* to remember us in a positive light, so the game is handicapped in your favor. Prepare the most moving eulogy about yourself you can imagine – then live it.

Day 17 Precious Moments

A wise investment ...

Every moment today will be a memory tomorrow. So, today, consciously make good memories. Pay close attention to each moment today, and consider how you can make it something you will enjoy looking back on. Then, at the end of the evening, think back over the day and take stock of the memories. What was good? What could have been better? It doesn't matter how well you think you did. It's the paying attention that matters.

Purposely creating positive experiences each day can be thought of as depositing currency into your memory bank for tomorrow. We all know we need to manage our money; but most of us never think about managing our moments. But we should. Because the only way to build a rich life – is one moment at a time.

Day 18 Anonymous

Kindness is its own reward ...

Make today a random act of kindness day. *Except,* look for kindnesses you can do that others won't know about. Pick up a piece of trash on the floor at the grocery store. Sure, it's somebody's job, but you just made that job easier. Do something for your partner that will make their life better, and don't tell them. Use your imagination. It doesn't have to be anything big. Everything is meaningful.

See how each small act makes you feel. And see how you feel at the end of the day. Yes, we all like to get credit, and that's important too. But anonymous acts of kindness are an often-overlooked source of joy. Take advantage of it.

Day 19 Mistakes

A list to make you laugh ...

Here's a great way to put mistakes into perspective and practice being fully present at the same time: Pay attention to the smallest details of your day, and catalog each time you "make a mistake." It's best to just keep a mental list, because you'll find in short order that *every day is full of them.* They're just so small and inconsequential, we don't notice. The following is a necessarily abbreviated list of examples:

You misplaced your keys. You can't find your phone. You forgot an appointment. You can't find your wallet. You sent a text to the wrong person. You forgot your password. You can't find your glasses. Consider also: Why do pencils have erasers? Why do they give us spare keys? Why do napkins exist? I could go on, but you get the idea.

The truth is, we make more mistakes in the first few hours of the day than we can count. And yet, on most days we don't even notice, considering them just part of everyday life. *Which they are.* Life itself is a constant optimization process, and mistakes are the guideposts by which we optimize – nothing more.

So, go ahead and make your mental list of screw-ups today. Keep it light. Just include the small ones. When you start laughing at them, your job is done. Then enjoy your new perspective. It will take a lot of the pressure off.

Day 20 Hi Mom!

A conversation …

If you could have a conversation with someone who has passed, who would it be, and what would you say? Look at it as a hypothetical conversation if you wish, or a real one, as it suits your belief system. But either way, it's a powerful conversation to have, because it will lead you down the road of gratitude, or of forgiveness – either of which is a beautiful road. If you enjoy the first conversation, expand the list and have them regularly. It will keep your soul healthy, and give you a larger perspective on the human experience. And they're never really gone, anyway.

Day 21 An Opportunity
Create your future …

Think of something you want. Be specific, and be definite. And then think only positive thoughts about it. How would it make you feel if it had already happened? See it in your mind's eye as already having happened. And don't accept any negative thoughts about it, or diminishing thoughts about yourself. Be consistent. Think about it in this way whenever it comes to mind, not just today. And then see how it makes you feel, and see what happens. Is this usually how you do things, or is this something different? What if we really do create our future? Be willing to spend some time on it. Most find the process of being specific about what they really want more challenging than they expected. Keep working at it. It will pay great dividends.

Day 22 Frustrated

A call to action ...

Make a list of things that frustrate you, and divide the list into three columns: Potentially Changeable, Unchangeable but Manageable, and Unchangeable and Untenable. Then think of things that frustrate you and put them into each column. It can show you a lot about your life that you may not have noticed.

Being continually frustrated over the same things is about lack of awareness more than anything. The list will help you see things in a different way. At the end of the day, it's an action list, remembering that making peace with things is an action too.

Day 23 Am I Smiling?

A list to brighten your day ...

Make a list of things that make you smile. You can list as many as you like, but a medium list is best. Too few on the list means you haven't spent enough time with it; and if there are too many, the list loses its power. Somewhere around ten is good. It can be a person, an event, a memory, or a future event; the options are endless. Just notice if it makes you smile; then, put it on the list.

To go deeper, try to prioritize the list as to which ones make you smile the most. This will be hard to do, but it is worthwhile because you'll smile even more as you try to make impossible choices. Don't worry too much about the order; it's the process that's the main thing, and the most fun. Make sure to write your list down, and refer to it often. There will be days when you'll need it (see Day 14).

Day 24 A Troubling Memory
Through different eyes ...

Think back to a troubling childhood memory. Is there another way to look at it? This isn't to deny that it happened, or that it was hurtful. Just realize that the emotion you feel when you think of it now, is compatible with the phase of life you were in when the event happened. So, looking back through adult eyes, things may seem different. Spend some time on it. Give it time to expand. Trying to see the same memory through other eyes at the scene is often helpful. Talk to your siblings if it's appropriate. It can be enlightening to see how differently people remember things.

Day 25 Disappointed

Broaden your perspective ...

Write down some things in your life that left you disappointed. And then consider some good things that came out of them. It may take some connecting the dots, but those things are always there. Often, even *great* things come out of them. Take the time to mentally find them, and it will take a lot of the sting out of things you may have lost; as well as infuse some hope into the next time you *are* disappointed. Make a short list, and refer to it when needed. It will lift you up when you are discouraged.

Day 26 A Long-Overdue Goodbye

Healing your past …

Take one of your troublesome childhood memories and actively go back and change the memory. No, you can't change the past, but you can imagine what it would have been like if it had happened differently. And if you imagine it vividly enough, it will shift your mental pathways to a new and more positive place. This is the power of imagery. Most use it to create a new future, but it can also be used to *re-create* a troublesome past. It is a seldom-used aspect of imagery, but considering its power and utility, it shouldn't be. It can truly set us free. It usually takes a little time for the images to evolve, so be patient with it. It will be worth the wait.

Day 27 The Magic Flute

Expand your life ...

Is there something you've always wanted to learn, but just haven't yet? This is something that could easily be done, but perhaps something you've put off. It could be learning a musical instrument, or a new language, or simply a new skill. It could be learning to do everyday skills with your non-dominant hand; just because it's an interesting challenge. Even this creates new brain pathways. And new brain pathways result in new perspectives, regardless of what stimulated the new pathways.

Life is so grand; and there are so many possibilities. Live it to its fullest, while you're here to do so. You won't be here forever. Take today and consider ways you can expand. Because when we expand in *one* area, we expand in *all* areas, in often imperceptible ways. No matter what you choose to learn, it's always worth the effort.

Day 28 The Inner Critic
Taking charge ...

We all have an Inner Critic, and even if you don't hear its voice right now – you will. So, it's good to prepare ahead of time. The main thing to remember is that you are in charge of your own mental space. *You* are the owner, and the Inner Critic is the unwanted guest, pretending to have something of value to say (it doesn't). Remember, it has no power over you until you believe what it tells you– so don't. The following is an exercise I have found helpful.

Since I want to put the IC in its place with a minimum of conversation, I have created a series of text shortcuts to send its way when it calls to me. It's playful, keeps everything light, but still gets the message across; "I don't believe you." The following are some of my favorites, but feel free to make up some of your own. Make them as colorful as you like. I have others I didn't include here for obvious reasons.

INL:	I'm not listening.	JGA:	Just go away.
GBSE:	Go bother somebody else.	TBS:	That's (baloney).
YIC:	Yes, I can.	JWM:	Just watch me.
IDBU:	I don't believe you.	NW:	No way.

Have fun with it. Keep it light. Laughter is a healing emotion. Your Inner Critic *hates* it – which should tell you all you need to know.

Day 29 Graduation Day
Finding your purpose ...

Consider why you are here, having this human experience. Admittedly, it's sometimes hard to know, but give it some thought. What is your life purpose? Most people feel they have one; they just don't give it much thought. Here's a hint: It's something you love doing. It's something that benefits others. It's something that may come to you so easily, you might not recognize how talented you are at it. When you do it, time seems to stand still. And you always feel uplifted afterward.

It may take some thought, but it's worth the time. But don't *over*think it. It could be as simple as a waiter pouring a bottle of wine with such presence that it's remembered years later. Each of us has a unique gift to offer the world. Find out what yours is, and start giving it away. It is the path to a joyful life – and the world is waiting ...

Day 30 The Rest of the Time
A life-changing connection …

Contemplate your connection to the Unseen Realm today. What do you believe about it? What, if any, is your relationship to it? What would you *like* your relationship to be with it? Give it some honest thought; because what we *say* we believe, and what we actually believe, are sometimes two different things.

Assign any name to it that feels right to you, but it's probably better not to name it at all, since this can get our left brains involved in this very right-brained activity. Explore the Unseen in any way that feels right. Asking questions is a good place to start; even if it's, "Is there anybody there?"

Day 31 A Labor of Love

It's good to reflect …

Take today and celebrate all the work you have done so far. If you've reached this point in the reading, and have been through all the exercises, your work has been substantial. Congratulate yourself for saying yes to the process. Not everyone does.

Any Day and Every Day
Because it bears repeating…

Of all the written exercises and meditations in *any* book, any*where*, the one that will benefit you the most is the practice of gratitude. It *is* that simple – because gratitude will bring you everything you want. It gives you a larger perspective, opens your heart, and expands your mind. Being grateful for something is like telling the Universe, *"I want more of this."* Finding gratitude can take some mental effort, depending on your mood. But the moment you find it, it begins to *lift* your mood. Yes, sometimes it's work, but so is digging for gold, or climbing out of a hole.

There are different levels of gratitude, ranging from **intellectual gratitude**, which consists of brief thankful thoughts for a person, thing, or event; to **heartfelt gratitude**, a physical sensation, usually felt in the chest; to **gratefulness**, an expansive experience of "at-oneness" where the sense of self fades, and there is a profound awareness of the interconnectedness of all things – which, when you get right down to it – is the whole point of everything.

As examples of the gratitude spectrum, consider the following excerpt from my book, *Journey to Hope*:

"Being grateful for your job, family, and a roof over your head will get you started…When you are grateful for butterflies, running water, rainbows, and toothpaste, you're on your way. When you are grateful for every breath, knowing that the next one is not guaranteed, you have arrived."

Simply put: Gratitude is *magic*. Live in it as much as you possibly can. Make it your *primary* goal in life; and it will help you achieve *every* goal in life.

A Parting Gift

Having now read this book, you and I are connected in a way that will never change, no matter where we go, or what we do. And not only are you connected to me, but also to everyone who has, *or ever will* read this book. And, with that in mind; as a parting gift to everyone who has shared this journey with me, I would like to offer this simple blessing to each and every one of us, based on the well-known Lovingkindness meditation:

May we be happy.
May we be healthy.
May we be whole.

May we be kind.
May we be forgiving.
May we be compassionate.

May we be bold.
May we be brave.
May we be powerful.

May we bring healing to ourselves, and to the world.

May we be wise.
May we be resolute.
May we be resourceful.

May we know, and live our purpose.

May we be abundant.
May we live in harmony.
May we live in love.

And may the world rejoice that we were here.

Acknowledgments

I want to thank my wife, Lana, for her love and support, and for taking care of so much in the background, which allows me to do what I love. Thank you to my grown children for being a lifelong source of joy. Thanks to April, Heather, and the team at O'Leary Publishing, not only for making this possible – but for making it so much fun.

Thank you to all the radiology technologists and nurses I have worked with. The relationships I've had with you have made the job so much more meaningful. Heartfelt teamwork is a beautiful thing – even if it's behind the scenes. And a special thank-you to Ingrid, who somehow knew I would write this book decades before I even knew. Your constant encouragement, both personally and professionally, has meant more than you know.

A special thanks also to the staff of Women's Center of Orlando, especially Susan, Vicki, and Michael. You were a crucial part of my professional journey. Your friendship wasn't part of the contract – but you gave it anyway. And I'm grateful.

Thanks to Gary, my first real spiritual mentor. And to his wife, Sandy, who preserved many of my early writings. I owe a deep debt of gratitude to you both. And thanks to Cathee and Sue for your love and support, and helping to make my previous book a reality. It made this one *so* much easier.

And thank-you to all the unnamed people who have been an inspiration in my writing journey. From a dear friend in the early days, without whom, there would *be* no writing, to all those who have encouraged me along the way – I owe a debt of gratitude to you all.

A special thank-you, also, to Dr. Jim Gordon, and the Center for Mind Body Medicine. The work you do has profoundly affected me, both personally and professionally. It has changed the way I look at life, and at myself. It literally has changed everything. And I am deeply grateful.

A special thank-you also to Nathan, my yoga teacher, who is always encouraging us to "find the profound in the simple." Your influence on this book is greater than you know. It makes me smile whenever I think of it…

And last but not least, thanks to Mom and Dad, where it all started. It's hard to overstate the importance of a stable home, and parents that are always sacrificing for you. *Thank you* seems like too shallow a term for all that you did for me. But it's all I can offer. Somehow, I know it is enough.

About the Author

Dr. Tom Hudson is a conventionally trained diagnostic radiologist specializing in breast imaging. He obtained his MD at the University of Maryland in Baltimore, and completed his radiology residency training at Walter Reed Army Medical Center in Washington, DC

After his time in the military, he settled in Naples, FL, where he served as Director of Women's Imaging at Naples Diagnostic Imaging Centers (NDIC), and later, as Women's Imaging Director for the entire NCH Healthcare System. He has also been honored as Doctor of the Year at Naples Community Hospital.

Dr. Hudson has always had a holistic view of health, and is the author of *Journey to Hope*, a book encouraging breast cancer prevention through a healthy diet and lifestyle. He is also on the faculty of the Center for Mind-Body Medicine (CMBM) in Washington, DC. Dr. Hudson believes that regardless of the surface ailment, true healing always begins from within. He currently works from his home office in Naples, practicing telemedicine, and providing online consultations via his website at thomashudsonmd.com.

www.ingramcontent.com/pod-product-compliance
Lightning Source LLC
Chambersburg PA
CBHW041323110526
44592CB00021B/2805